GOOD HEALTH
WITH
VITAMINS
AND
MINERALS

A COMPLETE GUIDE TO A LIFETIME
OF SAFE AND EFFECTIVE USE

JOHN GALLAGHER
Foreword by Dr. Brian L. G. Morgan

SUMMIT BOOKS
NEW YORK LONDON TORONTO SYDNEY TOKYO

Summit Books
Simon & Schuster Building
Rockefeller Center
1230 Avenue of the Americas
New York, New York 10020

SUMMIT BOOKS and colophon are trademarks
of Simon & Schuster Inc.

DESIGNED BY BARBARA MARKS
Manufactured in the United States of America

1   3   5   7   9   10   8   6   4   2

Library of Congress Cataloging in Publication Data

Gallagher, John
Good health with vitamins and minerals: a complete guide to a lifetime of safe and effective use / John
Gallagher ; foreword by Brian L. G. Morgan.
p.   cm.
1. Vitamins in human nutrition—Handbooks,
manuals, etc.   2. Minerals in human nutrition—
Handbooks, manuals, etc.   I. Title.
QP771.G35   1990
615'.328—dc20   89-22007
CIP

ISBN 0-671-66098-5

This book
is dedicated to
Elda Luisi,
the essential
supplement for
Good Health.

ACKNOWLEDGMENTS

Books are often collaborative efforts. This one is no exception. It was suggested, sponsored, edited, proofed, and corrected with the help of others. But the special efforts of Dominick Abel, Hugh Howard, Dr. Brian Morgan, and Dominick Anfuso made the book possible. I would also like to thank Charles Cole for his always helpful comments.

ACKNOWLEDGEMENTS

CONTENTS

PART III MINERALS 141

PART IV ISSUES OF ABSORPTION 233

FOOD TABLES 241

FOREWORD

Over the last thirty years, the importance of preventive medicine and the role of nutrition in good health has been recognized by health professionals and the general public. It has been clearly established that a poor diet contributes to most diseases and especially to the major, so-called killer diseases—cardiovascular disease, cancer, and diabetes.

More than twenty years ago, it became apparent that there was a link between diet and coronary artery disease. A high blood cholesterol level predisposes a person to heart attacks. Specifically, a diet high in animal fat, rich in cholesterol, will increase the blood cholesterol level in most people. Even people who have a family history of coronary disease (many of whom die from their first heart attack in their 30's and 40's) could have benefited from preventive measures. If these people with a high genetic risk had their cholesterol levels measured in their teens or earlier—as is the current practice for families with a history of coronary disease—they could have taken steps to reduce their dietary animal fat and cholesterol.

Furthermore, high-fat, low-fiber diets have been implicated in various kinds of cancers. A high intake of both vegetable and animal fat occurs in populations that show a high incidence of breast, endometrial, cervical, and testicular cancers. It is believed that the high fat intake somehow creates an imbalance of sex hormones that causes the cancer. A high-fat diet is also associated with colon cancer, especially if the diet contains little indigestible fiber. The excess fat increases the secretion of bile acids that are needed to digest and absorb the fat. But the bile acids also form mild cancer-causing substances when converted by bacteria in the large intestine. Reducing the amount of fat in your diet decreases the number of these low-level carcinogens in your intestine. The indigestible fiber found in vegetables, grains, nuts, and cereals also helps because they sweep up more of the bile acids and cancer-causing substances, reducing the amount of time they remain in contact with the wall of the intestine.

Another dietary problem is alcohol. Recent studies have shown that regular alcohol consumption, even in small quantities, may contribute to the risk of breast cancer.

Another disease affected by diet is diabetes. A direct link has been made between obesity and diabetes. Most diabetics develop the disease in middle age after becoming overweight. With 40 million people in the United States 20 percent or more over their ideal weight, it should not be surprising that there are so many diabetics in this country.

But obesity predisposes individuals to more than just diabetes. In the past two decades it has been conclusively linked to other problems, such as cancer, gallstones, heart disease, and hypertension. It was this correlation between disease and excess weight that prompted the National Institutes of Health to declare obesity a disease.

There are many thousands of proposed cures for obesity ranging from "miracle" foods that are supposed to change your metabolism, to claims for mechanical devices, such as belts and various massaging devices that will make it easy to exercise away excess pounds, or harmful liquid protein diets, to name but a few. None of these is an effective way to lose weight and keep it off. Weight reduction takes a balanced diet and exercise regimen that is designed for the steady loss of two or three pounds a week. While it is natural to look for easy solutions, the general health rule is if it took a year to put on the weight, it may take as long to take it off.

The consequences of a poor diet, especially one deficient in many essential nutrients, cannot be corrected by an indiscriminate use of vitamin and mineral supplements. At the same time, there are many occasions when nutrient supplements, even in excess of the RDA (recommended daily allowance), are helpful. For example, calcium supplements of 1,500 milligrams a day can be of great benefit, especially for the elderly who are at risk for osteoporosis, a serious bone-weakening disease.

There are other instances where nutrition supplements can be helpful, but the profession of nutrition has its fair share of quacks and one must be careful when wading through the many nutrition theories. For example, it is irresponsible to encourage people to take megadoses of most vitamins arbitrarily. This is often wasteful and occasionally harmful. High doses of vitamin B6 can cause irreversible nerve degeneration and megadoses of vitamin D can exacerbate hardening of the arteries. For some people, a belief in megadoses of vitamins and other supplements will give false hope of benefit and often lead them to disregard the medical advice of their own doctors.

These alternative therapies often rely on scare tactics to develop a reputation. Substances such as caffeine or food additives are singled out and condemned as harmful to your health with little or no scientific backing. Caffeine is a minor stimulant, and taken moderately, is not harmful. Often, a condemning charge is leveled at food additives, yet without many of them it would be impossible to get all the food needed to feed the American population from the farm to the table. As for the putative harm of food additives, nothing is added to foodstuffs until it has been extensively tested by the Food & Drug Administration. (Food additives do not cause cancer and are rarely implicated in hypersensitivity in children.) However, those people who have known allergies to specific additives should avoid those foods containing them.

It would be unjust to say that the food industry is adversely affecting the nutritional value of our food supply. Taste may have suffered for the sake of appearance, and we may yet come to regret the use of certain pesticides in the production of some of our food. But the fact is that the quality of food available to the average citizen has improved tremendously over the years. Vitamins and minerals lost in processing are routinely replaced in many foods, such as cereals and orange juice, and other foods are enriched with nutrients that are not normally present. One example is the current trend to introduce oat bran into processed and baked products. Oat bran has been found to reduce some people's blood cholesterol level by as much as 20 percent when those individuals regularly consume cereal containing at least 20 to 30 milligrams of oat bran.

The Federal Government continues to play a generally helpful role in establishing guidelines for the protection of our food supply and providing nutritional information and data for the healthcare professional and the public at large. One excellent example is the RDAs, or the Recommended Dietary Allowances, established by the Food and Nutrition Board of the National Research Council (NRC) in 1943. The RDAs, based on data from different population groups and ages, represent the average amount of a particular nutrient needed each day for various groups of people. Since actual needs differ by individual due to genetic differences and current needs, RDAs intentionally exceed the requirements of most people. For example, the NRC determined what amount of iron would meet the needs of more than 90 percent of adult women and added 30 percent to set a standard of 18 milligrams per day. Every five to eight years, the NRC reviews current scientific literature on vitamins and minerals and makes any changes deemed appropriate. Historically, certain nutrient levels have been increased with the publication of each successive RDA list. For example, the latest figures show an increase from 800 to 1000 milligrams in the calcium RDA for adult women.

Since the RDAs are a product of statistics, they do not address individual needs and must be used only as a guide. Exceptional nutritional needs may arise due to disease, surgery, or the use of medications that alter the way our bodies handle essential nutrients.

The RDAs should not be confused with the FDA's nutritional standards for labeling purposes, referred to as the USRDAs or Recommended Daily Allowances. This list, which appears on the labels of many processed foods and vitamins, tells what percentage of the USRDA for each of nineteen essential nutrients is contained in each serving or dose. The USRDA of any nutrient is the single largest amount required by any category of people in the American population, with the exception of pregnant and lactating women, based on the Recommended Dietary Allowances.

The nutritional education of the public is a serious matter and should be directed by responsible, well-informed individuals. Physicians would be the ideal people to convey this information, but they receive little education in this regard in medical school. Dieticians and nutritionists with degrees in nutrition from recognized university programs are perhaps the best sources of information at this time. If you do not have a special nutrition-related problem, however, such practitioners are an unnecessary expense. The information you need can be obtained from a guide such as this one.

Following a good diet can become habit-forming. You will lose your taste for fatty and overly sweet foods in time and learn that it is easy to prepare and enjoy healthful foods. Following a moderate exercise regimen will also be worth the effort. These simple changes in life-style will make us all look better, feel better, and probably live longer.

Dr. Brian L. G. Morgan,
Institute of Human Nutrition,
College of Physicians and Surgeons,
Columbia University

PREFACE

*G*ood Health with Vitamins and Minerals does not propose to offer easy answers, or all the answers regarding nutrition. What this book provides is basic information about all the vitamins and minerals essential to good nutrition, along with the key recent research that may affect your understanding and choices concerning their value and use for you and your family.

PART I discusses individually the special nutritional issues that are important to the needs of adult men and women, children, the elderly, and pregnant and lactating women.

The issues of nutrition for any one of these groups are broad and encompassing; therefore, we can only touch upon some of the more important concerns in Part I. (Specific data on all these issues and more are found in each of the entries devoted to the individual nutrients in Parts II and III of the book.) But each of these essays will heighten your awareness of how important nutrition is at every stage of life, and how nutritional needs change with age. Remember that what you knew then may not be applicable now.

PARTS II and III are the heart of the primer. They consist of individual chapters on each vitamin and mineral, opening with a brief summary of key information: the principal uses of the nutrient by the body; the best dietary source of the vitamin or mineral; those groups of people most at risk of a deficiency; recommended dosage (RDAs), including "Upper and Lower Limits of Dietary Supplemental Use"; both benefits and unproven benefits claimed for the nutrient; and any possible toxic symptoms.

What follows these summaries is a more detailed look. Most entries begin with a history of the nutrient's discovery, followed by sections devoted to its various functions and responsibilities in the body: specific problems related to having too little or too much of it; who might be at risk of a deficiency and why; information about various food sources and how nutrients are lost in many of these foods on their way to the kitchen and dinner table; some tips on how to protect the nutrient value of these foods during food preparation; and, finally, some pertinent information about those prescription drugs that might block the effectiveness of the nutrient.

PART IV provides general information about the processes of digestion, metabolism, and nutrient absorption, including how successful absorption of many nutrients is dependent upon the work of other nutrients. It also includes some key Food Tables, easy-to-use listings of dietary sources of vitamins and minerals complete with serving size and the amount of each nutrient in a serving.

Read from cover to cover, this primer will correct or enhance much of what you understand and believe about nutrition. It is more likely, however, that you will read those pages that deal with your particular questions and concerns and those of your family. As a result, we suggest that you read the relevant essays in Part I, and then browse through the entries in Parts II and III, paying special attention to key nutrients cited in Part I. As with other reference works, one of the dividends of a random reading of Good Health with Vitamins and Minerals is the discovery of a fact about one nutrient while pursuing another.

Of course, good nutrition is not found in a good book on nutrition but in a good diet. And so our wish is that you not only take to heart what you read in this primer but that you take it to your stomach, too.

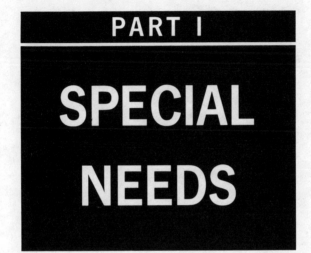

PART I

SPECIAL
NEEDS

CHILDREN

The quality of an infant's nutrition for the first twelve months of life can affect its health for years to come since nutritional needs are at their greatest during this remarkable growth period. A healthy infant's birth weight may double within the first four months—and triple by age one. So extreme is the growth that if a child were to continue to grow at that rate, the child would weigh 1,700 pounds by age four. In reality the average four-year-old weighs about forty pounds.

The first-year growth performance is so dramatic, then, that any failure to meet growth norms are considered decisive indicators of nutritional inadequacy and general health problems. The simplest way to know whether your baby is maintaining proper growth is to consult a growth chart. If the growth corresponds to the right percentile, then the baby is growing at the correct rate.

The seriousness of a problem with the child's growth rate that is created by a nutritional deficiency will depend on the age of the child when the deficit occurred and how long it lasted. Most serious problems concerning infant nutrition are prevented because inadequacies are detected early and corrected. If for any reason the nutritional problem is not rectified relatively early in the life of the child, however, the consequences could be permanent.

The success of a newborn's diet depends on the choice of early feeding method, when and how the child is introduced to solid food, and if the growth and nutritional status of the baby are carefully monitored. Infant feeding habits have changed over the years. Today, many pediatricians and nutritionists have differing opinions as to the best way to feed an infant. But experience shows that healthy infants do well with a variety of feeding practices.

INFANTS

Breast-feeding in the United States was an almost universal practice at the turn of the century. Then, in the 1920s and 1930s, many mothers adopted bottle-feeding, particularly women on the upper end of the socioeconomic scale. And by the end of World War II bottle-feeding was the choice of more than 75 percent of the mothers in this country.

There are several reasons, both cultural and medical, why American mothers abandoned breast-feeding practices. After World War I medical care moved more and more from the home into the doctor's office and the hospital. In particular, birthing moved out of the home and from the care of midwives and into hospitals where mothers were introduced to the newest ideas regarding prenatal and postnatal care. One of those new ideas was bottle-feeding. Another factor that may have influenced infant feeding practices was that nutritional science was able to produce a baby formula that appeared to be as healthful for the baby as their mother's milk. These two events coincided with a general movement of women into the workforce and their greater economic and social freedom. It was the bottle that freed many women from the confines of a nursing schedule.

In the past two decades, however, the medical community has thoroughly reviewed the relative merits of breast-feeding versus bottle-feeding. As a result, a growing number of healthcare authorities have begun to urge women to choose breast-feeding. The United States Surgeon General has found the evidence so compelling that he has made it a goal to have 75 percent of all babies breast-fed upon discharge from the hospital by 1990. Today, the percentage of women who choose breast-feeding has risen to over 60 percent.

But not only are more women choosing to breast-feed their infants, they are doing so for a longer period of time. Twenty-five years ago only 12 percent of mothers breast-fed their babies for the first six months, whereas it is estimated that more than 25 percent do today.

Breast-feeding has the following advantages:

1. The nutritional composition of human mother's milk is far superior to cow's milk. It is the standard against which healthcare professionals judge the nutritional value of all infant formulas.

2. The antibodies in the mother's milk give the child a natural immunity to many illnesses and possibly confer a resistance to allergies.

3. The trace elements in maternal milk are more readily absorbed by the infant because they are water soluble, whereas in cow's milk they are stored in fat. Vitamin D, which is usually stored in fat, is water soluble in mother's milk.

Nonetheless, many mothers still prefer bottle-feeding because of its convenience. Most working mothers find it difficult to arrange their schedule so they can find the time and place to nurse their child in comfort. Other mothers find nursing physically uncomfortable, even painful. Still others consider it not socially acceptable.

For whatever reasons mothers may choose not to breast-feed their babies, there exists a safe and sensible alternative in commercially prepared baby formulas. Most infant formulas are based on cow's milk, although soy protein is also used as a milk base, especially for those infants who develop a sensitivity to cow's milk. The infant is not fed whole milk but a "formula" that has been modified to meet the needs of the infant. To make it more acceptable to the infant, cow's milk is diluted to reduce the amount of salt and protein per volume, and more lactose is added so that there is the right amount of carbohydrate per volume. (Lactose is a sugar found in cow's milk.)

Essential vitamins and minerals are added, and the saturated fat of cow's milk is replaced by unsaturated (vegetable) fat which is easier on the infant's digestive tract. Heating the milk makes it easier for the infant to absorb its protein and reduces the likelihood of allergic reactions. In all respects, today's baby formula has been designed so that the infant is at no nutritional disadvantage if its mother chooses to bottle-feed rather than nurse.

SOLID FOODS There are different views as to when solid food should be introduced into an infant's diet. In the early 1900s pediatricians urged mothers not to feed their babies solid foods until they were at least a year old.

In the 1920s doctors began recommending broth at nine months, and in the 1960s many pediatricians urged mothers to try cereal foods as early as four to six weeks and solid foods by five months. The most recent wisdom is to recommend that an infant be fed only milk for the first six months. This does not reflect any new understanding of an infant's nutritional needs but rather the belief that a child over six months old can make the transition from milk to solid foods more easily than a very young infant. This transition should always be gradual; neither breast- nor bottle-feeding should be discontinued abruptly.

Some nutritionists and pediatricians also state that overfeeding children can occur by introducing solid food to infants who are too young to communicate when they have had enough to eat. Since excessive weight gain early in the life of the infant may have long-term consequences, it is considered prudent to reserve solid foods for the second six months of a child's life.

The first solid foods or strained foods are usually fed the infant with a spoon and a cup. These baby or junior foods are 70 to 90 percent water and contain primarily calories in the form of starch. Only after the infant has grown comfortable with these should real solid foods, especially those foods containing meat and fat, be introduced into the diet.

By the eighth month a child will usually eat cereal, mashed vegetables, egg yolks, fruit and fruit juices, and some pureed meat, and may also be learning to chew on bread or toast. A child this young should not be fed any other foods from the family table; foods such as raw carrots, nuts, and hard candies can easily cause the young child to choke.

During the second year of life, children can and should be encouraged to eat most solid foods. This change in diet will often cause a loss of appetite, but this is to be expected as the children make the transition from dependence to independence concerning what they do and do not want to eat. This temporary loss of appetite is called *physiologic anorexia*.

Older preschool children (four to six years of age) will continue to develop their own food preferences and, as with adults, their diet should be as varied as possible to ensure that they receive all the nutrients they need. It should include two to three cups of milk daily; one egg three times a week; about three level tablespoons of beef, lamb, poultry, pork, or fish each day; one or two servings of vegetables; plenty of fruits (especially citrus fruits because they are the only natural forms of concentrated vitamin C); and enriched cereals and breads. The distribution of calories in the diets of children should be from the same balance of food sources needed by mature adults: 7 to 15 percent should be derived from protein, 35 to 55 percent from fat, and the balance from carbohydrates. Children have significantly greater needs for most vitamins. (The RDAs for infants and children for all the vitamins and essential minerals are listed under the individual nutrients in Part II.)

It is well-known that everyone should eat a nutritious breakfast, but this is especially true of school-age children. Their lunches should provide at least one-third of their daily nutritional requirements. Because of their very active life-style and the rate at which they expend energy, the between-meal snack is an inescapable fact of life among school-age children. In most cases snacks do not affect a child's appetite, especially if eaten two or more hours before meals. It is quite clear that snacks are an integral part of the daily energy needs of most children, so unless it is apparent that they are negatively affecting their appetite, snacks should not be forbidden. You can, however, try to ensure that your child eats nutritious snacks, particularly fresh fruits and nuts.

Children between the ages of five and ten grow more slowly than they do in infancy or adolescence. During these years children will typically gain about five and a half pounds a year until the onset of puberty, when they begin a new period of accelerated growth.

ADOLESCENTS

A surge of biological changes and growth during the teenage years makes new demands on the nutritional life of adolescents and young adults. For males, this will be nutritionally the most demanding time of their lives; for females, only pregnancy and breast-feeding will require higher concentrations of essential nutrients. Both boys and girls often do not get enough vitamin A during their teenage years (a dislike of vegetables probably explains this phenomenon), while their intake of protein and niacin, which parallels their meat consumption, is generally adequate.

Boys and girls do have slightly different nutritional needs during adolescence. Teenage boys require more calories and vitamins A, E, thiamin, riboflavin, niacin, and protein than do girls. But the most significant nutritional difference between boys and girls during adolescence is not in their needs but in their eating habits. After the age of twelve, the diets of boys improve or remain stable whereas the diets of many teenage girls actually deteriorate as they move through their adolescent years, partly because of peer pressure which dictates that skinniness is more attractive than healthiness. To avoid getting fat, many teenage girls stop consuming milk and dairy products, leading to calcium deficiencies. They frequently go on and off diets and skip meals, sometimes to compensate for indulging in something "fattening." During a time when teenage girls need high levels of nutrients, both for growth and to prepare for their reproductive years, their diets are often highly inadequate.

WEIGHT PROBLEMS   Obesity is another serious health issue as it carries with it an increased risk of illness and death from a number of diseases including heart disease, hypertension, stroke, and diabetes. The problem of adult obesity in this country has brought some attention to the problem among children. Studies conflict as to the importance of early weight history. Most overweight infants (ages 1–3) do not become overweight adults, but preadolescent obesity does appear to have a strong correlation to adult obesity.

Some practical measures can be observed against the problem of excess weight in children: (1) Breast-feed if possible. (2) Do not overfeed. (3) Do not use food as a reward. (4) Urge children to be active unless restricted by the child's doctor. (5) Do not place the child on a diet unless supervised by a pediatrician. Weight loss is not a suitable practice for children, and any diet that falls below 1,400 calories may compromise the child's growth. A stable weight is more important because it allows them to grow normally.

Excess weight isn't always in the adolescent's imagination. One out of every three teenagers is overweight and as many as one out of every ten is obese (20 percent over their recommended weight). Generally, this is due not to excessive food intake but to a lack of proper exercise, especially for many teenage girls.

Whatever the reasons for excess weight, adolescence is a good time to develop a workable weight control program that includes exercise and sensible eating habits since weight retained through adolescence often leads to adult weight problems.

Recent studies have determined that there are probably two types of obesity: Type I is a condition in which the fat cells grow too large; Type II is a condition in which there are too many fat cells. What is meaningful about their difference is that these two conditions require different weight reduction techniques to achieve the same weight loss.

The most important fact to understand is that weight reduction reduces only the size of the cell; it does not reduce the number of fat cells. As a result, an obese person with Type I obesity can reduce the size of each fat cell to its normal size and have the same amount of fat tissue as a thin person.

On the other hand, an obese individual with a Type II condition has to reduce the size of the fat cells to below normal in order to have normal fat tissue because they have a greater number of fat cells. The Type II obese person will have a far more difficult time both losing weight and keeping it off because that person must maintain less fat in each fat cell than even a normally thin person.

The discovery of Type II obesity makes clear that preventive measures must be taken during the two critical periods when an increased number of fat cells may develop: infancy and adolescence. Although excess weight gained during infancy or in adolescence may create an abnormal and permanent number of excess fat cells, this is no reason to place slightly overweight children or teenagers on strict or low-fat diets because fat cells are necessary to support their most dramatic growth period. If you have concerns about the weight of your child, you should consult your pediatrician.

Far more serious than obesity for teenage girls is a disorder known as *anorexia nervosa*. More than a hundred years ago an English physician, Ernest Gull, named this disorder of voluntary starvation to describe severely emaciated young women who refused to eat. Anorexia nervosa affects girls who tend to be high achievers, above-average academically, and usually fairly gregarious with many friends. They are also very interested in health and exercise. (This profile is quite different from the bulimic person—see page 27.) Today, nearly one in every 250 girls between the ages of twelve and eighteen is affected by anorexia nervosa. This disorder is rare among boys.

The underlying psychological causes are complicated and not always easily treated, but if successful treatment is not provided early, the anorexic may suffer from muscle loss, osteomalacia (softening of the bones), and amenorrhea (a delayed or suppressed menstruation).

Anorexia nervosa begins with an obsession with thinness, which may lead to a 25 percent loss of weight. An anorexic teenager will become ineffective in school and occasionally hyperactive, and will often complain of discomfort after eating. Many anorexics also go on a strict regime of exercise in an effort to lose more weight, even though they are eating less and less.

Because their diet is usually very soft with few, if any, foods with natural fiber, they develop constipation. This occasions the use of laxatives; but laxative abuse, which reduces nutrient absorption, often becomes part of the disorder, too. (Constipation will continue to be a worsening problem if the disease is not treated.) Due to a profound and long-lasting protein deficiency, the muscles of the digestive tract grow weak. Eventually the gastrointestinal tract starts to waste away. The narrowed and weakened digestive tract further discourages the child from eating bulk foods because they make her progressively more uncomfortable.

The chronic anorexic will develop unmistakable signs of protein starvation: anemia, frequent infections, and an irregular heart rate. The endocrine and immune systems will begin to dysfunction. If untreated, the patient will fall into a coma. One out of twenty anorexic patients dies, but the majority of them are treated successfully and "grow out" of their disorder.

Anorexia nervosa always requires professional treatment. You should not treat a child with this disorder yourself. The child should be encouraged to eat, without regard to what is eaten, and should not be fussed over whether or not the diet is balanced. Professional treatment consists of discovering and solving the underlying psychological problems and restoring normal food intake and consequent weight gain.

Bulimia is another eating disorder that affects teenage girls. Also known as the binge-and-purge disorder, bulimics will go on eating binges in which they might consume between ten thousand and twenty thousand calories, then purge themselves by inducing vomiting or taking laxatives. Following a binge-and-purge episode, the bulimic may fast for days. Understandably, bulimic girls experience frequent weight fluctuations.

Unlike anorexics, bulimic girls appear to be of normal weight and tend to be somewhat older. Bulimic girls generally are depressed (the principal drug for treatment is an antidepressant), secretive, and ashamed. They may also have trouble controlling other impulsive behaviors, such as promiscuity, shoplifting, alcohol and drug abuse.

Only half of the bulimia patients fully recover. About 25 percent live with some symptoms most of their lives, and another 25 percent never recover from the disorder at all. Bulimia may be fatal because the persistent vomiting can produce a serious imbalance of electrolytes. Potassium depletion, specifically, can cause the heart to stop (see page 164).

Both eating disorders are caused by a complex web of psychological, social, and biochemical factors. Bulimia does not last more than about two years with teenagers, but among older patients the disorder may last six years or more. Early intervention is the most effective way to deal with both anorexia and bulimia.

Often, adolescents know more about nutrition than is reflected in their eating habits. Nonetheless, bad eating habits are a product of a rapidly changing life-style and the pressures of peers. Fortunately, most young people grow out of these more serious eating habits that pose a health risk.

It is advisable to give your teenager or recommend to your college-bound child a one-a-day vitamin and mineral supplement. This does not replace the need for a balanced diet, but it will ensure that the child is receiving the Recommended Dietary Allowances of vitamin and minerals. Most anorexics take vitamins since they are usually very health conscious; however, if they are not taking a multivitamin and mineral supplement, it is strongly recommended. The same is true for someone suffering from bulimia. But there is no vitamin/mineral therapy for the treatment of either one of these disorders. They both require professional help.

ADULT MEN AND WOMEN

Over the past seventy years our growing understanding of nutritional chemistry and dietary deficiencies has resulted in the virtual elimination of diet-deficient diseases in this country that plagued adults and children alike. Once it was discovered that inadequate amounts of specific nutrients in our diet were responsible for certain diseases, we varied our diets to include the missing nutrients or they were added to our foods. For example, the iodine-deficient disease of goiters was successfully treated by adding iodine to table salt; vitamin D was added to milk and margarine to guard against the risk of rickets. Yet we are still faced with a number of nutrition-related diseases: Six of the leading causes of death in this country—atherosclerosis, cancer, coronary disease, diabetes, liver disease, and strokes—are directly linked to our diets.

The reasons our diets pose potential health risks are related to both what we eat and what we do not eat. Our principal dietary problem is fat; most of us eat too much of it. The diet of the average American adult is 40 percent fat, which is 30 percent more than most nutritionists believe is necessary for good health. The diet of most American men averages between 700 and 800 milligrams of cholesterol per day, which is three times more than is needed.

Ideally, we should consume more of our calories in the form of complex carbohydrates because they are more easily metabolized and utilized in this form. Calories in the form of fat, on the other hand, are not easily broken down but are stored as fat tissue. In addition to increasing the risk of obesity, excess dietary fat predisposes us to certain types of cancer.

Another fact of our dietary life is that we eat too little of some foods. More precisely, many of us do not consume enough fiber. As a result, the problems associated with a low-fiber diet are on the rise, such as cancer of the colon and rectum. Less serious gastrointestinal diseases, such as frequent constipation and diverticulitis, are also related to a low-fiber diet.

Generally speaking, we do not consume adequate amounts of calcium. During the past thirty years, milk consumption has gone down, especially among women, and this decline in dietary calcium is believed to be partially responsible for the increased incidence of osteoporosis in our society.

Another mineral deficiency is iron. As many as 30 percent of the women of reproductive age in this country have less than the optimal intake of this mineral. Besides causing chronic fatigue and anemia, an iron deficiency can threaten the health of the unborn child during pregnancy.

Another deficiency in our diet is folic acid. This problem is especially widespread among young women, but many premenopausal women also have lower than adequate amounts.

The issue of good health is very much a matter of eating right. The best nutritional approach is still a balanced diet that consists of two servings of both milk and dairy products, and protein-rich foods, with four servings of vegetables and fruits, and breads and cereals.

OBESITY

One-fourth to one-half of all Americans are either overweight or obese. Obesity is another health problem for millions of Americans as it carries with it an increased risk of illness and death from diseases such as heart disease, hypertension, stroke, and diabetes. The federal government has classified obesity as a disease occurring in men whose body fat exceeds 20 percent of their total body weight (normal values are from 15 to 18 percent) and in women whose body fat exceeds 28 to 30 percent of their total weight (normal values are from 18 to 24 percent). While estimating percentage of body fat is a fairly simple procedure that is often carried out at health fairs, obesity may be judged more simply against ideal weights based upon height and bone structure (fine, medium, or heavy). Anyone weighing 20 percent or more over the ideal weight may be considered obese, with the exception of body-builders and other athletes who have acquired added muscle weight through weight-building programs.

HEALTH ISSUES Obesity has clearly defined health risks for adults. Those with a high percentage of body fat are likely to have abnormal amounts of fat circulating in their bloodstream, leading directly to cardiovascular disorders such as heart attack, stroke, and hypertension (high blood pressure). (Relatively thin people may also have high cholesterol levels.) An increasing amount of evidence points to a similar relationship between excess blood fat and cancer. The relationship between diabetes and obesity is not as clear-cut, but obesity is often an early sign of diabetes and a complicating factor in its development and treatment.

Many overweight women experience high blood pressure and diabetic symptoms during pregnancy. Overweight women are also more likely to develop postpartum infections that are not usually serious but require treatment. Osteoarthritis is also complicated by obesity though not caused by it; added weight may increase the discomfort of the sufferer and further damage weakened bones.

The reasons so many people have trouble maintaining a desirable weight can range from genetic factors to metabolic disorders to their own psychology. The solution is not always more exercise and less food. There is convincing evidence that some overweight people actually eat less food than those who have no problem controlling their weight. It may be that obese people metabolize their food more efficiently, converting more of it to stored energy in the form of fat. They may also be less able to mobilize or withdraw the stored fat for current energy needs. Consequently, for many obese people, weight control is a struggle that goes well beyond simple willpower.

One theory has it that at a set point the body begins to defend itself against further loss of fat by sending out signals that suppress appetite and change the rate of metabolism to maintain this ideal weight.

Eating habits are important in the attempt to understand obesity. For both conscious and unconscious reasons, many obese families make more food available—more is served, and it is served more often. They are also more likely to consume large quantities of food at night when food is stored as fat for use at a time of lower intake or increased need.

DIETS AND DIETING

Obese people are usually more concerned with how much they are eating than with whether they are eating a balanced diet. The grossly obese (40 percent over their ideal weight) usually eat fairly nutritious foods. It is not true that they usually binge on sugary snacks of "junk" foods or are fat primarily because of such a diet. The real nutrition issue for them is how they can reduce the total amount of calories they consume.

But most people are not grossly obese. In fact, many of the people who undertake weight-reduction diets are by definition not even obese. For reasons other than health, millions of Americans participate each year in a weight-reducing regimen. The weight-reduction business, which includes programs and diet aids (products), has become a $10 billion industry in this country. But despite this devotion to weight loss and weight gain, the public is still remarkably misinformed about some basic nutritional facts.

One area of our nutritional ignorance is reflected in the kinds of fad diets we continually embrace and then abandon. A fad diet is one that is not based on sound nutritional principles. It is usually marketed so that its promises of easy weight loss catch the public's eye. Aside from exaggerated claims, the fad diet is frequently not balanced nutritionally. A common trait is that it emphasizes only one or a few foods such as fruit. As we all should know, fruit does not contain adequate protein, vitamins, and minerals for normal body functioning. Equally discouraging is that surveys consistently reveal that within a year of starting a popular fad diet 95 percent of all participants are unable to sustain their weight loss.

Then what is a good diet for adults? Apart from helping someone steadily lose a reasonable amount of weight, it should provide all of the nutritional needs for a healthful life while offering the probability of lasting success. Such a diet should:

• establish a reasonable reduction in caloric intake. Cutting 500 calories from your daily diet makes you lose a pound each week. It should be noted that in the first week of a high-protein, low-carbohydrate diet you tend to lose a lot of water from your body. This occurs because a low-carbohydrate diet causes you to use up your body's glycogen that is stored in water several times its weight. As the glycogen is used, so is the water. During the first days of your diet, then, it is lost water that accounts for much of the initial weight loss. Consequently, during the second week your weight loss may not be as significant because your body will work to restore the water loss. You may even regain some weight. It should be noted that with the exception of extreme obesity, the weight-loss rate of a diet should not exceed more than 2 or 3 pounds per week; for example, a minimum of two months should be allotted for someone wanting to lose about 20 pounds.

• include foods from all major food groups. A diet of only 1,400 calories can still include at least two servings of milk and dairy products; fruits and vegetables; cereal products; meat, fish, and poultry; and eggs. If you must cut your caloric intake to under 1,400 calories, your doctor may tell you to take vitamin and mineral supplements to ensure that you get the correct amount of all essential nutrients.

• contain some fat and perhaps relatively high levels of protein. Fats and protein will postpone hunger pains longer than carbohydrates.

• be inexpensive and relatively easy to adapt to meals taken at home or in restaurants. The more difficult the diet is to follow, the more likely you will abandon it.

DIET AIDS Though some dieters feel the need for added help, diet aids are not usually essential to a weight loss program. They even undermine your own resolve, if you come to rely heavily on them.

CHOLESTEROL FAT AND DISEASE

The association of cardiovascular diseases with a high fat intake has been suspected since the early 1960s. But the link between dietary fat and heart disease has been accepted only since the late 1970s, and only in the last five years has it been established as a medical fact. (In many medical societies throughout the world, and especially in Great Britain, it is not yet accepted that a high fat diet causes heart disease.) In 1984 the American Cancer Society added cancers of the breast, prostate, and colon to its list of dangers of a high fat diet.

Cholesterol, a soapy-looking yellowish substance, is an important fat in virtually all animal life. Cholesterol is necessary for building cell tissue, for a healthy nervous system, and for the manufacture of sex hormones, among other body activities.

Cholesterol is both ingested with the food we eat and manufactured by the body. In both cases it is stored in the liver. When the liver reaches its maximum level of storage, the excess cholesterol is circulated through the blood system and deposited along the walls of the arteries. The thickening and loss of elasticity of the arteries caused by the cholesterol buildup is called atherosclerosis and is a primary cause of coronary heart disease.

The body is normally capable of regulating the total amount of cholesterol by reducing the amount it produces by approximately the amount that is consumed, as long as that amount is less than 150 milligrams daily. If more than that is consumed, our blood cholesterol levels begin to rise.

While the ideal blood cholesterol level is 180 milligrams of cholesterol per 100 milliliters of blood, not all of the many millions of people whose cholesterol levels are greater than that are at a significant health risk. Cholesterol levels as high as 212 for men and 230 for women are still relatively safe.

All dietary fats are not the same, however. There are three types of fat: saturated, polyunsaturated, and monounsaturated. The primary difference, for this discussion, is that saturated fat raises the level of cholesterol, while monounsaturated and unsaturated fats actually lower cholesterol levels. It is important that these three fats be maintained in relative balance. Nutritionists therefore urge us both to reduce our dietary fat consumption to 30 percent of our total caloric intake and to bring our consumption of saturated and unsaturated fats to a 1:1 ratio. Some nutritionists, knowing the history of our fat consumption, set a goal of 2:1. Still, most of our eating habits fall short of these recommendations. The ratio of saturated-to-unsaturated fat in the average American's diet is about 7 to 1.

The easiest way to reduce the excessive amount of these saturated fats in our diet is to eat less fatty meat and dairy foods such as cream and cheese. It will also help to avoid using butter and the fats of meats in cooking, and to steam, broil, boil, or stir-fry foods so that they absorb little or no fat in their preparation. (See page 246 for a table of the cholesterol content of selected foods.)

ORAL CONTRACEPTIVES

While important for family planning, oral contraceptives have nutritional side effects that must be understood if they are to be used safely. For reasons unknown, contraceptives cause a rise in the concentration of triglycerides and other fats in the bloodstream, resulting in the increased risk of a heart attack, stroke, or blood clot. As the concentration of those blood fats also increases with age, the health risks increase the older you are while using an oral contraceptive. Women with a history of blood clots, hypertension, severe diabetes, or breast or uterine cancer are urgently advised by physicians not to take the pill.

Less well known are some nutritional consequences of oral contraceptive use. Generally, they are not as serious as the aforementioned health risks, but they can be crucial to good health, depending on the woman's overall nutrition as well as on the length of time she has been taking the contraceptive.

Contraceptive use tends to deplete the body of riboflavin (vitamin B2), vitamins B6, B12, and C, and folic acid. In most instances if early signs of a deficiency develop (see each nutrient for early warning signs), a diet rich in that nutrient and a daily supplement of the Recommended Dietary Allowance (RDA) is usually all that is required. If the symptoms persist, however, see your doctor.

Vitamin B6: The estrogen hormone in oral contraceptives stimulates many reactions in the body that require vitamin B6. Since smokers appear to have an increased need for this vitamin, women who smoke while on the pill may increase their risk of a vitamin B6 deficiency as well. Oral contraceptive use may have some long-term effects on the body's ability to use vitamin B6. Generally, it has been thought that a woman's ability to use vitamin B6 is quickly restored to normal once she has stopped taking the pill. Some recent studies have shown, however, that breast milk was deficient in vitamin B6 in lactating mothers who had taken oral contraceptives as long as two and a half years prior to the onset of pregnancy. (See Lactation on page 39.)

This assault on vitamin B6 may explain why some women report that they become depressed while on the pill. The hormone serotonin, produced by the brain, elevates our mood. The production of this neurotransmitter depends on another vitamin, B12. A woman's vitamin B12 and B6 levels would have to fall very low to seriously affect serotonin production, but it is possible, given the fact that probably 50 percent of Americans consume only two-thirds of the recommended amount of vitamin B6.

Vitamin B12: Estrogen reduces the absorption of vitamin B12, technically increasing the likelihood of a vitamin B12 deficiency; however, it is rare to develop a B12 deficiency due to oral contraceptive use alone. Deficiencies are more frequently caused by an underlying malabsorption problem or a diet especially poor in B12. One example is a strict vegetarian diet combined with use of the pill. (See Vitamin B12, page 115.)

Vitamin B2 (riboflavin): Just as estrogen reduces the absorption of vitamin B12 because of accelerated metabolic functions, it also increases the need for riboflavin. A dry cracking of the skin in the corner of the mouth is a common sign of a deficiency in any or all three of these vitamins.

Folic acid: Oral contraceptives also seem to hamper the absorption of folic acid. The diets of one out of three women in this country are already poor in folic acid, and as many as 7 percent suffer from anemia caused by a folic acid deficiency. (See Folacin, page 126.) All women, but especially those on the pill, should make sure that they are getting enough folic acid in their diets. That is to say, they should be eating plenty of leafy green vegetables. If not, a daily supplement of 400 micrograms of folic acid may be advised.

Vitamin C: Women who use oral contraceptives metabolize vitamin C more quickly than those who do not, which means that if you are on the pill and your intake of vitamin C is marginal, you could develop a modest deficiency over time.

Alcohol: Heavy drinking is always ill-advised but especially so for women taking birth control pills. Oral contraceptives slow down the metabolism of alcohol so that it stays in the body longer, making it far more likely to accumulate toxic levels. Alcohol can also be a problem because, like the pill, it impairs the absorption of vitamin B6.

Oral contraceptive use can also increase appetite, which accounts for weight gain that occurs for many women on the pill, especially during the first year of its use. The pill may also enhance the stimulating effects of caffeine.

It is highly unlikely that you will ever develop a serious vitamin deficiency due to oral contraceptive use alone, but combined with a poor diet, four or five years on the pill may deplete you of several of the vitamins you need. There are no specific vitamin supplements that exist for women on the pill. If a woman were to become pregnant shortly after coming off the pill, however, her body might be depleted of folic acid to some degree. As a safety measure, this woman should take folic acid supplements.

PREGNANT AND
BREAST-FEEDING MOTHERS

A mother requires quality nutrition before, during, and after her pregnancy. During her pregnancy she must provide all the necessary nutrients the developing fetus needs for proper growth. If she chooses to breast-feed, she must be able to produce enough milk to nourish her child, whose nutritional needs will change before and after birth. A woman who has looked after her own nutritional needs before she conceives a child begins her pregnancy with a reserve of nutrients that helps her meet the needs of an infant without jeopardizing her own health. If she is not well nourished at the outset of her pregnancy, however, her own health may suffer because the developing child often gets first call on the nutrients available.

A mother's body goes through a series of physiological changes to help meet the nutritional demands of a pregnancy. A series of changes in body chemistry, signaled by the production of hormones that support the pregnancy, improves the metabolism and absorption of certain nutrients such as calcium and iron.

The placenta is a mass of tissue embedded in the wall of the uterus through which the exchange of nutrients and waste products takes place. The placenta also produces hormones that control the metabolism of the fetus and sometimes of the mother. Later in pregnancy the fetus also receives some of the nutrients through the amniotic fluid.

During the first trimester the fetus gains little more than 1 gram of weight every day and needs little in the way of nutrients. During this period, however, good nutrition is crucial to the development of the placenta and amniotic fluid, the growth of breasts and uterus, and the expansion of the mother's blood supply. The placenta of a poorly nourished mother is less able to aid in the flow of nutrients from the mother's bloodstream, screen out toxics, and produce needed hormones for the metabolism of the fetus.

During the first trimester many women experience nausea or morning sickness. It is not clear why this intestinal distress occurs, but it is speculated that it may be caused by the stress of establishing the relationship between the fetus and the mother. Another view is that it is brought on by the high fat levels in the blood. Many pediatricians recommend smaller meals of carbohydrates during this period. There is no evidence, however, that vitamins will cure or relieve nausea during pregnancy.

During the second trimester the mother's nutritional task is to store fat. This serves as insurance against the possibility that the mother may not be able to provide all the food needed by the fetus in the coming months, and it also acts as a reserve of energy for the strenuous task of nursing after the child is born.

By the beginning of the third trimester the fetus gains about 10 grams daily and is using most of the mother's intake of nutrients. Half of the fetus's total weight increase takes place during the last two months. It is especially important, therefore, that a mother's diet be unusually rich in foods that provide high-quality proteins, minerals, and vitamins during the final months of pregnancy.

THE PREGNANCY DIET   In addition to a well-balanced diet of a mix of dairy products, eggs, meat, whole grains, nuts, beans, and vegetables, pregnant women should increase their intake of dairy products to two glasses of milk daily; fish, poultry, and beans; and dark leafy green vegetables. They should also consume at least one egg a day and plenty of fruits and vegetables, to provide a surplus of the vitamins and minerals needed by the growing fetus.

Calcium, iron, folacin (folic acid), and zinc are often missing in many diets and are especially important during pregnancy. These nutrients are discussed in detail in later entries (see Calcium, page 147; Iron, page 189; Folacin, page 123; and Zinc, page 208, but it should be noted that the best source is your food because they appear there in balanced quantities. Since many nutrients, and especially B vitamins, function interdependently, any excess of intake of one will create a deficiency of another. An imbalance is possible if they are taken as individual supplements. In some instances, however, an obstetrician may recommend a prenatal vitamin and mineral supplement as a safeguard.

During pregnancy a woman's need for niacin may increase 15 percent (see Vitamin B3, page 99), and her need for folacin may double. Energy needs increase as well—by as much as 15 percent. A diet that emphasizes high-density nutrient-rich foods can meet most of the increased demand for essential vitamins, minerals, and other nutrients while keeping calorie intake within reasonable limits. An example of a high-density nutrient-rich food is milk; another is fish. They are rich in nutrients while containing relatively few calories. On the other hand, a candy bar may contain many calories with relatively few nutrients. This kind of food is often referred to as empty calories. It may be very difficult, however, for some women to maintain a diet high in nutrients over the 280 days of pregnancy without gaining more weight than needed. Multivitamin and mineral supplements can be of help in these instances.

According to the Food and Drug Administration (FDA), nutritional supplements for pregnant women should provide between 50 and 150 percent of the RDA for the following vitamins and minerals: A, D, E, K, thiamin, riboflavin, B6, B12, C, folacin, calcium, iron, sodium, iodine, magnesium, and zinc. The FDA provided these standards because vitamin and mineral supplements not explicitly intended for use in pregnancy often contain too much of some elements and not enough of others, and they include some unnecessary nutrients while lacking essential ones. You should discuss with your doctor whether you need supplements and which supplements you should take during pregnancy.

RESTRICTIONS Pregnant women are sometimes advised to restrict their intake of salt, but this is usually necessary only in cases of excessive weight gain or swelling due to buildup of tissue fluid known as *pathological edema*. As for caffeine, the jury is still out, but most physicians advise their patients to cut down on coffee consumption while pregnant.

LOW BIRTH WEIGHT BABIES As many as one out of every seven babies born in this country weighs less than 5½ pounds, a condition referred to as LBW, or low birth weight. About 70 percent of these babies are underweight because they were born prematurely, after fewer than thirty-seven weeks of gestation. LBW babies born after forty weeks of gestation are usually the result of the mother's poor nutrition during pregnancy.

All LBW babies are at a risk for several health problems: They are more susceptible to infections, may have difficulty metabolizing carbohydrates and proteins, their kidneys may not be fully developed, and frequently they have trouble regulating their body temperatures. Consequently, these babies are far more likely to be hospitalized during their first year than babies of normal weight.

Teenage mothers are more likely to give birth to LBW babies because they still have significant nutritional requirements for their own growth. Premature and LBW babies are also more likely to be born to mothers who during their pregnancy gained too little weight (less than 16 pounds) or too much weight (more than 30 pounds), smoked more than half a pack a day, or drank heavily.

LACTATION

Though breast-feeding mothers may feel they no longer have to "eat for two" following their child's birth, the fact is that lactation is even more nutritionally demanding than pregnancy. Within four months a healthy breast-fed baby will double the weight gained over the entire nine months of pregnancy. Thus, its mother's milk during these months must contain more energy in the form of calories than was required during the entire pregnancy.

The American Academy of Pediatrics has long advocated breast-feeding, stating emphatically that mother's milk is the best food for every newborn infant. In general, breast-fed children are healthier and better able to resist infection than bottle-fed children, who are far more likely to have respiratory and intestinal infections. Bottle-fed infants are admitted to the hospital nine times as often as babies who are breast-fed.

Breast-feeding benefits the mother as well. During a normal pregnancy she will store approximately thirty-five thousand calories of fat for future milk production. Nursing mothers generally find it much easier to return to normal weight after pregnancy. If she doesn't nurse, however, she will have to lose about 10 pounds on her own. Recent statistics also reveal that breast cancer rates are lower among women who have breast-fed a child before the age of thirty. After thirty, breast-feeding has no statistical significance.

The quantity and quality of the nutrients a mother has stored during the last months of the pregnancy to support her milk production do not depend solely on her current diet. If her diet is poor in calcium after her baby's birth, her own calcium stores will be used to maintain the calcium quality of her milk. (See Calcium, page 147, for a further discussion of calcium and maternal milk.) Nor are all of a baby's nutrients stored in its mother's milk. Nearly a six-month supply of dietary iron, copper, and other essential minerals consumed during pregnancy is stocked in the child's liver. Not all essential nutrients, however, are stored in advance. If vitamins A, E, B6, and thiamin are deficient in a lactating mother's diet, they will be deficient in her breast milk as well.

Also, oral contraceptives taken for more than two and a half years prior to conception can reduce the amount of vitamin B6 in breast milk. Lactating women who took oral contraceptives shortly before becoming pregnant may require supplements of 2.5 to 5 milligrams of vitamin B6 per day to compensate for the lack of the vitamin in their milk.

THE LACTATION DIET   The diet for a nursing mother resembles that recommended for pregnancy except that nutrients are needed in greater quantities as the child begins to take more and more milk. This means a well-balanced diet of dairy products, eggs, meat, fish, fruit, whole grains, nuts, beans, and vegetables. After pregnancy many women overlook fruits and vegetables, yet these not only supply many needed vitamins and minerals but also help replace fluid lost in lactation.

Increased calcium and phosphorus needs are best met by a quart of milk a day. The diet should include cheese and yogurt, too. If you have an aversion to milk or dairy products and your doctor recommends supplements, they should be taken at bedtime and shortly before nursing the baby.

Many obstetricians suggest a multivitamin and mineral supplement for lactating women, but they should avoid other kinds of supplements, many of which contain insignificant amounts of some essential nutrients and excessive amounts of others. High doses of some vitamins, such as vitamins A and B6 which can pass directly into the infant's milk, may cause serious problems. Supplements can never replace a good balanced diet, however, which provides the fiber, protein, and many trace minerals not generally included in supplements.

Some lactating mothers choose to avoid beans, cabbage, onions, and garlic for fear that they will give their child gas or colic. It is not likely, but for reasons unknown, beans can produce flatulence in some sensitive breast-fed infants. Other women do not drink carbonated beverages. Again, carbonated drinks pose no threat to the baby's health, but it is thought that excessive consumption of beverages with the sweetener aspartame could possibly disturb the baby's sleep. There is no harm in eliminating these foods from your diet, but there is little evidence that these foods will cause any problems in breast-feeding infants except possibly in the very sensitive.

Plenty of exercise, fresh air, rest, and an adequate and satisfying diet will enable most healthy mothers to nurse their infants comfortably and to mutual advantage throughout the first six months of their children's lives.

THE ELDERLY

Aging is a process marked by change. In the past we have largely ignored how many of these changes—physical, physiological, and psychological—affect the nutritional needs of the elderly. Through the efforts of the National Institute on Aging and the USDA laboratory at Tufts University, and other organizations, however, we are now beginning to understand more about how nutrition influences body functions during the aging process.

It is well recognized that the average diet of the older population in this country does not meet RDA requirements. There are many reasons for this inadequacy, including the loss of physical powers that makes it more difficult for many elderly people to shop for, prepare, eat, and digest nutritious foods. By the age of seventy we lose about two-thirds of our taste buds, and therefore many people take less pleasure and interest in food. Also, many drugs, including diuretics, will decrease sensitivity to taste and cause a loss of appetite. The elderly also secrete less gastric juice, which makes digestion take longer, in many cases reducing the number of desired meals each day. Depression, a common problem among the elderly, also influences appetite. Some respond to their depression by overeating, others by undereating; both pose nutritional problems.

Obesity is more of a problem among the elderly than among the general population, perhaps because many people continue with long-standing food habits despite more sedentary lives. It is two to three times as prevalent in older women as in older men and is directly related to the increased incidence of diabetes among the elderly.

Meanwhile, people who take their meals alone tend to eat less and more erratically than those who eat in the company of others. For many of the elderly the social aspect of meals is important not only to combat loneliness but to aid good nutrition. Also, as we age our cells become much less able to utilize the nutrients available. Absorption of essential nutrients may decrease by as much as 40 percent.

Our hearts and lungs function less efficiently, circulating essential nutrients much less effectively. Because the heart pumps less blood, it is filtered through the kidneys half as often. As a result, the kidneys filter less waste and recapture and reabsorb fewer nutrients. With age comes a reduction in liver bile, which helps in the breakdown of fats, and a decline in hydrochloric acid, which aids in the utilization of protein and the absorption of calcium, and iron.

Aging also reduces the ability of the lining of the stomach and the intestines to generate new cells, which impairs the absorption of many nutrients, such as iron and calcium. The chronic intestinal diseases, and folacin and protein deficiencies, common among the elderly, impair absorption, too.

HEALTH PROBLEMS RELATED TO NUTRITION

Not all the factors that affect nutrition among the elderly are directly related to aging. As in younger people, diseases and other health problems affect their nutrition. Many of the elderly are affected by the nutritional consequences of the many prescription drugs they take to treat various ailments.

More than 30 percent of all prescription and over-the-counter drugs sold in this country are purchased by people over the age of fifty-five. Many of these drugs directly or indirectly affect the way our bodies handle essential nutrients. Digitalis drugs, prescribed to improve the strength and efficiency of the heart, generally cause some loss of appetite. Diuretics, frequently prescribed to the elderly for the treatment of high blood pressure, can deplete the body of zinc, calcium, potassium, and magnesium, as well as thiamin (vitamin B1), which may already be in short supply in those with a high-carbohydrate diet. Steroids, used to treat inflammation, are widely known to impair the absorption and utilization of calcium, protein, potassium, and vitamins B6 and C. Virtually all anticancer drugs are highly nutrient antagonistic. (*Note:* Each entry in this book has a listing—Drug Interactions—that identifies those drugs that reduce the effectiveness of the nutrient.)

OSTEOPOROSIS   One of the most feared problems of the elderly is taking a fall and breaking a hip. Osteoporosis is a disease of the bone in which the bone loses its store of protein and calcium (and some other minerals), causing it to become weak and porous. (In Greek *osteon* means bone and *poros* means passage.) Nearly a quarter of a million people, most of them over the age of fifty-five, break their hips each year due to osteoporosis. Both men and women lose bone mass steadily after the age of thirty-five: Women may lose as much as 1 percent of their total bone mass per year; men about half that much. This can be attributed to a low intake of calcium, phosphorus, and/or protein; poor absorption of calcium in the intestine or reabsorption in the kidneys; or poor production of the active form of vitamin D (normally found in the kidneys). Osteoporosis is not a selective disease; the fact is that the older you become the more bone mass you will lose. However, calcium intake that falls below 450 milligrams daily, a sedentary life-style, small bones or slight build, a family history of osteoporosis, and use of steroids, anticonvulsants, anticoagulants, or the heavy use of antacids increase the risk of severe osteoporosis. Women are likely to be affected after the age of fifty; men after the age of seventy. Black men and women are less likely to be affected than white men and women. (See Calcium, pages 150–51, for a more extensive discussion of this disease.)

NUTRITIONAL NEEDS OF THE ELDERLY
Information about the specific nutritional needs of the elderly is still very incomplete. While the RDA lists different requirements for three-year age groups of adolescents, they provide only one set of requirements for people age fifty-one and over, ignoring the different nutritional needs that may exist among people in their sixth, seventh, and eighth decades. These differences may be as pronounced and distinctive as those in the various stages of adolescence.

CALORIES Calorie demands differ widely among the elderly depending upon health, age, and level of activity. Many older people either eat too much or too little, however, and most do not eat enough protein or get enough iron. Many cling to old eating habits formed when their nutritional needs were quite different; for example, many neglect milk and dairy products, which they need to supply them with calcium, vitamin B12, riboflavin, and other nutrients. Some also avoid meat, perhaps because meat is expensive and difficult to chew, thus reducing their iron intake. Those who avoid both milk and meat often suffer from a lack of vitamin B12, one of the two most common causes of anemia among the elderly. (The other is a shortage of iron.)

On the other hand, many diets contain too much phosphorus, which probably reflects a diet that heavily favors meat and soft drinks. The problem with a high phosphorus diet for the elderly is that it increases their already high risk of a calcium deficiency.

VITAMINS   Vitamin C, which is needed to help absorb dietary iron, is a common deficiency among the elderly, perhaps because, like meat, citrus fruits are expensive and can be difficult to chew and swallow. In an effort to lose weight, many older people eliminate potatoes from their diet and lose an inexpensive source of vitamin C (and other valuable nutrients).

Folic acid is one of the most common nutritional deficiencies among all ages, but especially among women and the elderly. Often when older people are depressed, chronically tired, or experiencing circulation problems, they are seriously deficient in folic acid. (See Folacin, page 123, for a further discussion of this nutrient deficiency.)

Riboflavin (vitamin B2) and niacin (vitamin B3) deficiencies are rare, but vitamin A levels are often low among the elderly, probably because their diets are short on dairy products and vegetables. A lack of vitamin D may become a problem for those older people who rarely spend time outdoors. The ultraviolet rays of just twelve minutes of sunlight convert enough of the provitamin substance in the skin to activate vitamin D to last for the day. The housebound should drink vitamin D-fortified milk or eat canned salmon, herring, or sardines to compensate for the lack of sunlight. (See Vitamin D, page 61, and Calcium, page 147, for a further discussion of this problem.)

Many of the elderly do not drink enough water. Water needs vary, but all adults should drink at least two quarts per day, as tap water or other beverages. (See Water, page 181, for an expanded discussion of a necessary but largely forgotten nutrient.)

An understanding of the special nutritional needs of the elderly means understanding some of the various changes age will bring to all of us. If you are over the age of fifty-five, be reminded that a balanced nutritious diet can also be an interesting diet; it can be a diet that allows for any practical difficulties you may have and satisfy the eating preferences you have formed over the years. Finally, the diet that cannot meet your nutritional requirements should include a one-a-day supplement of vitamins and minerals.

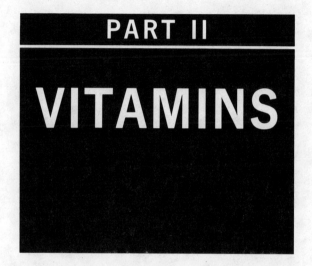

PART II

VITAMINS

Since childhood we've been told that nutrients are essential to good health and that a balanced diet would provide all that we would ever need, but the fact is that most people don't consistently eat a balanced diet. Our diet doesn't always provide the right amount of fats, carbohydrates, proteins, vitamins, minerals, or other micronutrients that we need.

While a less than perfectly balanced diet may not pose a threat to our daily health, it could do so whenever our need for nutrients increases. Specific illnesses, surgery, pregnancy, aging, and various prescriptive drugs make demands on our bodies for increased amounts of certain nutrients. If these are not readily available in our diets, we are at risk of deficiencies that may in the short run affect our energy level, cause cracks in our lips, give us a sore tongue or bloodshot eyes, or lower our resistance to infections; in the long run they may make us seriously ill and cause permanent damage such as a weakening of bones that leads to osteoporosis.

Even if our diet is consistently deficient or unbalanced, it does not follow that vitamin (or other nutrient) supplements are suitable food substitutes. Vitamins are not a source of energy, although there are probably millions of people who use them for this reason. Only the calories found in proteins, fats, and carbohydrates provide energy. Vitamins only help release the energy potential in our food, and only small amounts are normally needed for this job. Nutrient supplements only complement our diet—they don't replace it.

Yet supplements can compensate for certain, though limited, weaknesses in our diet. Consequently, an awareness of poor eating habits and an understanding of how various life changes make very specific nutritional demands on our diet appear to be the reasons for the extraordinary and widespread use of nutrient supplements in this country.

But not everyone agrees about the true value of supplement use. The traditional medical view has been that supplement use has very limited value and that nearly all of the claims of beneficial results from supplements have no scientific basis. On the other hand, the true believer in vitamin and mineral supplements often espouses, indiscriminately, near-miraculous results from supplements. These are the two extremes; the truth lies somewhere in between.

The professional healthcare community has come to believe that there are sound arguments in favor of the benefits of supplements. Nutritionists have come to accept that the diets of many Americans do not provide the optimal amount of vitamin and minerals to ensure good health. In the past decade they have also discovered other people who are in need of supplementation, such as patients recovering from illnesses or gastrointestinal surgery, or those who abuse alcohol and tobacco. For these reasons and because many people abuse the use of supplements, nutritionists have begun to advise people when and how to use them.

While the evidence grows in support of many of the claims made for supplement use, at the same time many popular claims have proven to be untrue. One popular myth is that natural vitamins are somehow superior to synthetic vitamins. The clinical fact is that no one has been able to adequately demonstrate that the body can tell the difference. Natural and synthetic vitamins perform the same functions, usually with the same level of efficiency. The exception may be vitamin E, which in synthetic form may be less potent. (See Too Much Vitamin E, page 71.)

When are supplements harmful and when are they safe? The Federal Drug Administration believes that almost one out of every ten persons who use supplements may be taking more than is safe. The levels of supplements considered dangerous depend on a number of factors, including weight, metabolism, diet, health, and nutritional status, as well as the form of the nutrient and how often it is taken.

The safest way to take supplements is to keep dosages of each nutrient to the limits designated by the RDA or within the limits of safe use that appear in each entry of this book. Millions of people regularly take megadoses (more than ten times the RDA) of vitamins and minerals, primarily because they don't understand the risks of exceeding safe levels of consumption. They have been led to believe that the greater the dosage, the greater the benefit. This is far from the truth. Supplements should be treated much as drugs are. If properly handled, supplements can be helpful; if abused, they can cause serious problems.

THE HISTORY OF VITAMINS   For centuries people have understood that some foods have specific qualities that made them essential to good health. As long ago as 400 B.C. it was known that calf's liver had properties that would cure night blindness. In the fourteenth century a popular verse assured everyone that

> If night blindness should befall,
> Liver of goats do not spurn,
> If enough of this you eat,
> Darkness into light will turn.

In the early eighteenth century James Lind, a Scottish naval physician, suspected that scurvy, a disease that plagued British seamen, was related to a poor diet. He suggested that sailors eat citrus fruit to combat the disease. His advice was ignored for forty years, but in 1795 the British navy began to include lime juice in the sailors' diet and the disease disappeared.

During World War I the Danish government shipped the country's entire production of butter to England and Germany for a substantial profit. The Danish ate margarine instead, and drank skim milk (the fat was skimmed off to make butter). As a result, the children in rural areas began to develop a disease of the cornea of the eye called xerophthalmia, or night blindness, in epidemic proportions. Once the government restricted the export of butter and the children began to receive their customary diet of fresh butter (which is rich in vitamin A), the disease virtually disappeared.

Thus, people have long known that there was a link between certain foods and the prevention or cure of various ailments. Until the twentieth century, however, they believed curative powers were unique to certain foods. It did not occur to them that liver's ability to cure night blindness was due to a substance that might be found in other foods, such as sweet potatoes. (Liver does contain substantially more vitamin A than any other food, which is how it got its reputation.)

THE SCIENCE OF NUTRITION

Before the turn of the century, good nutrition was thought to include carbohydrates, proteins, minerals, water, and some fat. People had little conception of the substances we call vitamins. It was only in 1912 that a Polish scientist named Casimir Funk, working in a London research laboratory, coined the term: Dr. Funk discovered that the hull from polished rice contained an organic-hydrogen compound, or *amine,* that prevented beriberi. (Years later this substance was identified as vitamin B1.) He named his discovery *vitamine*—combining *vita,* the Latin word for life, with *amine.* The *e* was dropped from his spelling in the 1920s when it became apparent that all vitamins do not contain the hydrogen compound amine.

But *vitamine* was not the only name used for these essential factors. At the turn of the century, scientists had isolated the macronutrients of foods—protein, fat, and carbohydrates. Sir Frederick Hopkins, a British scientist, established that rats would become sick and die if they were fed food composed of only these basic nutrients. On the other hand, if they were also fed just a small amount of whole milk (which contains vitamin D), they would survive. When Hopkins discovered this, he called these micronutrients missing from the pure protein, fat, and carbohydrate diet "accessory food factors," a term British scientists used for many years. In 1929 Sir Frederick Hopkins shared the Nobel Prize in medicine and physiology with a Dutch biochemist, Dr. Christiaan Eijkman, for their work in the field of the "vitamin concept." Dr. Paul Karrer, a Swiss chemist credited with first synthesizing a vitamin (vitamin A), received the Nobel Prize for his work in 1937.

Despite these and other awards, the credit for the discovery of vitamins must be given to a wide range of researchers working on the same problems in several countries. At about the same time Sir Frederick identified "accessory food factors," scientists working in different parts of Europe, America, and East Asia arrived at the same conclusion: Animals fed purified food would suffer various diseases and eventually die; but when fed whole foods and not just a mixture of the then-known constituents of food, animals thrived.

The scientific community reasoned that there must be a variety of unknown organic substances in some (or perhaps most) foods that were necessary to life, but they couldn't actually identify them until the 1930s when chemistry succeeded in establishing the chemical structure of carbohydrates, fats, proteins, and vitamins. Once they realized that foods contained substances critical to growth and good health, they were eager to isolate them and learn their chemical structures. Their method was to try to extract vitamins from foods in which they were reasonably sure the vitamin was readily available: vitamins A and D from fish oil; B vitamins from rice polishings and liver; vitamin C from citrus fruits and red peppers.

This work of extraction was not an easy task. Many of these vitamin compounds are so fragile that they are destroyed by exposure to heat or air. Furthermore, research required that the biochemists isolate substantial amounts of each vitamin from foods that contained only minute quantities. The actual vitamin content of food represents only 1 ounce in every 150 pounds of dried food.

Once extracted, these substances were concentrated and purified until what remained were small quantities of pure crystals. In its crystalline form, it was possible to identify the chemical properties and eventually manufacture synthetic vitamins in the laboratory. Synthetic vitamins not only made it easier and less expensive to conduct animal studies but also made it possible to enrich the vitamin content of certain foods. The cost of synthetic riboflavin (vitamin B2) is little more than twenty-five cents per 1,000 milligrams—more than a year's requirement for one person. Inexpensive synthetic vitamins also made it possible to fortify animal feed, which in the case of vitamin D permitted farmers to raise animals indoors year-round. (Pet food is also fortified with vitamin D.)

Government programs to enrich foods with vitamins and other nutrients began during World War II. In 1941 the FDA created the first program to enrich or "fortify" certain foods that had suffered some nutrient loss through processing or marketing. Fortifying some foods with ascorbic acid (vitamin C) can prevent the loss of other nutrients. Added nutrients also enhance the economic as well as the nutritional value of products such as vitamin-fortified snack bars and cereals for children.

The term "fortification" was originally used to describe the effort that replaced lost nutrients in foods, such as vitamin D in pasteurized milk and vitamin C in fruit drinks; "enrichment" is a legal term referring to the FDA program that requires thiamin, riboflavin, niacin, and iron be added to refined cereals. Fortification and enrichment are now used interchangeably, however.

NAMING VITAMINS When vitamins were first discovered, it was clear that they were not all the same. Initially, scientists saw that some were soluble in fat (for example, vitamins A, D, E, and K) and others in water (vitamins B1, B2, B3, C, folacin, pantothenic acid, and biotin). They also learned that some contained nitrogen and others did not. Most important, they realized that these substances performed different functions in the body. It was decided, as a practical matter, to give each new vitamin a letter of the alphabet, in the order of discovery. In the case of the B vitamin, however, it was learned after its initial letter was assigned that there were many B vitamins. As a result, they were designated B1, B2, B3, and so forth.

Vitamin K is another exception to this orderly alphabetic rule. A German-speaking Danish scientist discovered that a vitamin had to exist in some foods to explain blood clotting. It became known as vitamin K when it retained the *K* from the German spelling of its first name: koagulation vitamin.

This alphabetical naming procedure was abandoned when the chemical nature and structure of each vitamin was established. When the chemical structure of vitamin B1 was identified, it was given another name: thiamin. Vitamins B2 and B3 were designated riboflavin and niacin, respectively. The letter system has become so firmly established in the popular mind, however, that it is unlikely those vitamins first given letters will ever completely surrender the letter designations for their newer chemical names. Vitamins discovered after the 1930s (such as folacin, pantothenic acid, and biotin) have been given only chemical names.

Vitamins are necessary only in minute quantities for normal growth and maintenance of health. Still, the body is unable to manufacture most of the vitamins it needs. With the exception of vitamins K and B3, which can be produced in small quantities in the body, and vitamin D, which is also in the skin with the help of the ultraviolet rays of direct sunlight, all vitamins must come from outside sources in our diet.

Vitamins prevent certain diseases such as scurvy and xerophthalmia, the disease of the cornea mentioned earlier; but they are also responsible for maintaining a healthy appetite and digestive tract, and a healthy nervous system, and providing a general resistance to infection. Vitamins undergo a chemical change to form coenzymes. In this form vitamins accelerate specific metabolic reactions in the body and promote the proper utilization and metabolism of all the nutrients in our diet; for example, thiamin (B1) and niacin (B3) are needed to break down carbohydrates into a form of energy we can use.

Vitamins do not act independently of each other or of other nutrients; their work is collaborative. Vitamin E enhances the effectiveness of vitamin A, whereas too much vitamin E, combined with an excess of vitamin C, actually hampers the effectiveness of vitamin A. Some vitamins need certain minerals to be effective: Vitamin E, for example, relies on selenium, thiamin, and sulfur, while several B vitamins need phosphate. Several minerals need vitamins to be effective. Vitamin C aids the absorption of iron, and vitamin B12 helps iron function inside the body. Without vitamin D, calcium is unable to be absorbed and stored in our bones and teeth.

This cooperation among vitamins and minerals breaks down when any of these nutrients is present in excessive quantities. In other words, an overdose of one nutrient can create a deficiency in another. For example, an excessive intake of vitamin E impairs vitamin K, while too much iron decreases the effect of vitamin E.

As we have already seen, your vitamin requirements will differ at different stages in your life, but they also vary from person to person. Some adults require only two-tenths of a milligram of thiamin per day, while others seem to need four times as much. It is this consideration that prompted the National Research Council (NRC), who created the Recommended Dietary Allowances (RDAs) in 1943, to establish categories divided by age and gender, and to acknowledge the special nutritional needs of pregnant and lactating women.

The most common cause of vitamin deficiencies is a poor diet, though deficiencies can also result from poor absorption of nutrients or the increased need that comes with adolescence, pregnancy, lactation, or serious illness. When the rate of our body's systems is accelerated, as it is during a fever, we need more vitamins. People suffering from tuberculosis require more vitamin C, and alcoholics have an increased need for thiamin. Because estrogen stimulates many reactions in the body, most women taking oral contraceptives have a greater need for vitamins B2 and B6. People who eat either too little of certain foods like vegetables or dairy products or too little in general to provide them with the nutrients essential to good health are in danger of deficiencies, a problem complicated by the fact that modern harvesting, processing, and storage procedures encourage vitamin loss in many foods. Cooking also drains many foods of vitamins, especially the water-soluble B vitamins.

Since vitamins are organic, they are subject to being destroyed by exposure to heat, light, and oxidation. The length of time the food is stored and the amount of heat, air, or sunlight to which it is exposed will govern how much vitamin loss occurs.

Food preparation will always cause some vitamin loss, but more nutrients are lost or destroyed when foods are prepared at high temperatures; cooked in large amounts of water (and the water discarded) or in pans that expose a large surface area of food to the air; prepared with alkali (baking soda); or stirred or agitated during cooking. You can minimize vitamin loss by cutting food into small pieces for faster cooking, using a minimum of water and the lowest possible cooking temperature, keeping liquids just below boiling (to reduce agitation), and covering food to reduce cooking time and losses from evaporation.

Even if the vitamin content of someone's diet is entirely adequate, various absorption problems may lead to a deficiency. People who have difficulty absorbing fats also have difficulty absorbing fat-soluble vitamins. Some people who do not secrete enough of a protein, called "intrinsic factor," do not properly absorb vitamin B12. Someone recovering from gastrointestinal surgery may have general absorption problems. Though many people are just realizing the importance of fiber in their diets, too much fiber accelerates the passage of food through the gastrointestinal tract, reducing the time for proper absorption of essential nutrients.

There are two broad categories of vitamins: fat-soluble and water-soluble.

Vitamins A, D, E, and K are stored in the fat of your body and are generally found in fatty foods (the fats of meats and fish, butter, cream, and some vegetable oils). Vitamin K is stored in body fat but found in leafy green vegetables. Since fat-soluble vitamins are stored in quantity (a two-year supply of vitamin A is stored in the liver), a deficiency in any one of them is slow to develop and initially difficult to detect. The fact that these vitamins are stored also means that vitamins A and D can reach toxic levels if consumed in excess. For this reason one should never take supplements containing more than ten times the recommended dosage of vitamin A or D without consulting a doctor (see each nutrient entry for safe levels). High levels of vitamins K and E do not pose the same toxic threat, though too much vitamin E may interfere with the effectiveness of other vitamins.

Fat absorption problems also affect the absorption of fat-soluble vitamins. Obstructive jaundice and celiac disease interfere with the absorption of fat. These disorders, if not successfully treated, may lead to a severe vitamin deficiency.

Fat-soluble vitamins are not readily destroyed by heat or lost through exposure to air. As a result, fewer of these fat-soluble vitamins are lost during cooking or processing.

Unlike fat-soluble vitamins, water-soluble vitamins are easily dissolved in water and are not stored in the body. B complex vitamins, the principal group of water-soluble vitamins, are necessary to unlock the nutrients in carbohydrates, proteins, and fats, and convert them to available energy.

B vitamins are not all the same, however; they have distinctly different functions and characteristics. While some B vitamins help enzymes break down the food we eat, others help manufacture red blood cells. Supplements of B vitamins may be prescribed to treat infections, stomach problems, or herpes.

The members of this family of vitamins work in concert. To function properly, all the B vitamins must be present in specific ratios to each other. When that ratio is altered by a deficiency of one or an excess of another, all of them are impaired.

Current popular wisdom states that megadoses of water-soluble vitamins "can't hurt" because any unused excess is washed out of the body. This is not necessarily true. At one time it was thought safe to take vitamin B6 in almost any quantity. Now we know that megadoses of vitamin B6, over time, lead to permanent and irreversible degeneration of the nerves. Though quite rare, high levels of vitamin C in the blood have caused gallstones in some people. On the other hand, it is virtually impossible to reach toxic levels of nutrients from food sources only. The exception might be vitamin A because people could conceivably develop a toxic buildup of the vitamin if they were to consume vast quantities of carrot juice. There is little data available on the consequences of megadoses of vitamins (and other nutrients as well) because it is a relatively recent phenomenon, but as people continue to take anywhere from ten to one hundred times more than the recommended dietary allowance, we may learn more about the potential dangers.

VITAMIN A

DESCRIPTION

Vitamin A plays a number of important roles in the proper functioning of the human body. It is needed for the health of the outer skin and the body's inner lining. A pigment of the eye that is critical for night vision is dependent on vitamin A, and the vitamin supports the functioning of the respiratory and immune systems, aids in the growth of teeth, hair, and eyes, as well as the reproductive organs of women.

FOOD SOURCES

Excellent Sources: beef liver, sweet potatoes, pumpkin, carrots, cantaloupe, winter squash, broccoli, and apricots

Good Sources: peaches, whole milk, butter, asparagus, brussels sprouts, kale, spinach, mustard greens, tomato juice, yogurt, summer squash, green peas, corn, eggs, and green beans

RISK GROUPS FOR POSSIBLE DEFICIENCY

- pregnant or breast-feeding women
- teenage girls
- the elderly
- alcoholics
- people who have suffered from severe burns or wasting diseases
- people recovering from gastrointestinal surgery
- heavy users of Dioctyl Sodium Sulfosuccinate, a drug that softens the stool
- heavy users of Colestipol Hydrochloride (Colestid), a drug that lowers blood cholesterol and triglyceride levels
- heavy users of mineral oils or a drug called Sucralfate used to treat ulcers
- chronic use of antacids

RECOMMENDED DOSAGE

GROUP	RE*	IU	GROUP	RE*	IU
Pregnant women	1,000	5,000	Children 7–10	700	3,300
Lactating women	1,200	6,000	Children (females) 11–18	800	4,000
Infants 0–.6	420	2,100	Children (males) 11–18	1,000	5,000
.6–1	400	2,000	Adult women	800	4,000
Children 1–3	400	2,000	Adult men	1,000	5,000
4–6	500	2,500			

(RDA for vitamin A is expessed in retinol equivalents [RE], which is the term for the form of vitamin A commonly found in all the animals but not in plants and freshwater fish or birds that feed on them.)
(*Note: 1 RE = approximately 5 IU or International Units)

UPPER LIMITS FOR REGULAR DIETARY SUPPLEMENT USE

Children under 4 years of age: 2,500 IU
Adults and children 4 or more years of age: 5,000 IU
Pregnant or lactating women: 8,000 IU

BENEFITS

TREATING DEFICIENCY SYMPTOMS
- night blindness
- weight loss
- dry skin
- dental decay
- frequent respiratory infections

OTHER POSSIBLE BENEFITS
- aids in the treatment of acne, boils, and impetigo (when applied externally)
- helps maintain healthy hair

UNPROVEN BENEFITS (UNRELATED TO DEFICIENCY SYMPTOMS)

- reduces the symptoms of glaucoma
- reduces the effects of air pollution
- prevents skin cancer
- removes age spots
- reduces stress symptoms

TOXIC SYMPTOMS

Peeling and dry skin, dizziness, headaches, nausea, hair loss, joint pains, drowsiness, and extreme lethargy.

DISCOVERY   In 1913 Elmer Verner McCollum, an American biochemist at the University of Wisconsin, discovered that a factor essential to life was present in some animal fats. He called this fat-soluble substance "fat-soluble A." McCollum contributed to the discovery of other fat-soluble vitamins, such as vitamin D in 1922 and vitamin E still later, but his most notable discovery was this first vitamin.

Vitamin A was not only the first to be identified, but in 1931 it was also the first vitamin to have its chemical structure determined. This work was done by a Swiss chemist, Paul Karrer, who received the 1937 Nobel Prize in chemistry for synthesizing vitamin A as well as for synthesizing vitamin B2 in 1935.

ROLE   Vitamin A has been studied for almost sixty years, but the role it plays in our overall health is still not well understood with the exception of its function regarding our vision. The four distinct functions with which it has been identified are vision, growth, cell division, and reproduction.

The process of dark adaptation is one of the more dramatic examples of vitamin A function. Dark adaptation is required to adjust our vision when moving into dim light and when moving into bright light after leaving an area of darkness. The speed of recovery of vision in both instances is determined by the amount of vitamin A available to perform the transition.

Vitamin A is essential to growth, and researchers believe that aside from night blindness (poor vision in dim light), failure to grow is probably the next most likely consequence of vitamin A deficiency. It is believed that vitamin A is also essential for normal bone growth.

Vitamin A is required to maintain the growth of epithelial cells (found principally but not exclusively in the outer layer of the skin). It may also provide a broad protection for our immunological system as well.

Although the mechanism is not well known, studies with rats indicate that a lack of vitamin A appears to cause a failure of sperm production in male rats and the abortion of the fetus in female rats. On the basis of this evidence some nutritionists believe that vitamin A may be helpful to the reproductive systems of women.

PROBLEMS OF TOO LITTLE VITAMIN A   Vitamin A deficiencies, known as *hypovitaminosis A*, are widespread outside the United States, especially among children. The deficiency is not easily detected until it has become severe because the storage capacity of vitamin A in a healthy person is thought to be as much as two years. Nevertheless, when a vitamin A deficiency does develop, the symptoms can be dramatic.

Hypovitaminosis A can cause night blindness, damage tear secretion (an inability to tear), increased susceptibility to respiratory infections, dry or rough skin, poor bone growth and weak tooth enamel, weight loss and diarrhea, and it can stunt growth in children. An early sign of a vitamin A deficiency is often abnormally rough and dry skin and diarrhea because it affects changes in the lining of the gastrointestinal tract.

WHO IS AT RISK?   Nutritionists believe that most Americans receive an adequate diet of vitamin A, but there are exceptions, of course. Studies show that the diets of some teenage girls, pregnant women, and the elderly are deficient in vitamin A. These people should add vitamin A supplements to their diet. Others who are generally in need of more vitamin A are abusers of alcohol, people with wasting diseases or who have undergone surgery, especially for partial removal of the gastrointestinal tract, and patients who have suffered severe burns.

VITAMIN CONVERSION   Vitamin A is present only in animal foods, but it is not produced in the animal. The question, then, is where do animals get their vitamin A supply if they can't manufacture it? The answer is, of course, in their diet.

Many plants contain vitamin A, or more properly a substance known as *provitamin A carotenoid,* commonly known as carotene. The carotene is taken in by the animal (or human) and converted to vitamin A. The herbivore or vegetable-eating animal meets its need for carotenoid by grazing on green plants. The carnivore, which doesn't eat vegetables, sensibly eats herbivores (as prey) that have the carotene in their diets. In the case of fish, the larger fish eat smaller fish, and the smaller fish, in turn, eat yet smaller fish. In this manner the feeding reaches down through the food chain until it comes to the very small plankton or crustaceans that feed on marine plants.

PLANT SOURCES   Many plants contain provitamin A carotenoid, which is converted into vitamin A in the walls of our intestines. The plants that are an excellent source for this carotene are noted for their distinctive yellow or orange-yellow pigment: carrots, sweet potatoes, squash, pumpkin, apricots, peaches, and yellow corn.

The yellowish color, however, is not a foolproof method of identifying carotene plant sources. Researchers have also found carotene in dark leafy green vegetables as well. They rightly concluded that the yellow or orange-yellow pigment of the carotene was being hidden by the dark green pigment of chlorophyll.

STRATEGIES

FOOD SOURCES   Liver is the richest food source of vitamin A. Kidneys are also an excellent source. Vitamin A appears in the fat of animal foods as retinol. Consumed in this form the body converts it to vitamin A for its use. The significant difference between carotene and retinol is that retinol is about three times as potent. That is why liver, which is where the animal stores its vitamin A, is by far the best-known source of vitamin A. (See the food table on page 259 for a list of vitamin A-rich foods.)

The vitamin A value of certain animal foods will vary depending on how much vitamin A was in the animal's diet. It is believed that the liver from older animals and animals that feed on green fodder contains more vitamin A. The farmer will tell you that cows that graze in green pastures in the spring will produce a butterfat that is more yellow (carotene) than that produced when they are stall-fed in the winter. Thanks to improved cattle feed for dairy cows over the past twenty years, this seasonal variance in vitamin A values of dairy milk has been reduced, though not eliminated.

As the Vitamin A table shows, most of the foods are vegetables and some are fruits. Yellow-orange fruits and green vegetables dominate the list. Fruits such as apricots and cantaloupes are excellent sources, along with sweet potatoes. Among the green vegetables, vitamin A is produced in quantity in the thin green leaves of spinach, collards, kale, and other greens.

FOOD PREPARATION   Vitamin A is not as sensitive to heat as other vitamins, especially water-soluble vitamins. Fat-soluble vitamins such as vitamin A will not dissolve if boiled in water, nor will they lose their basic value when subject to ordinary cooking temperatures. (Carrots actually increase the amount of biologically available vitamin A when cooked.) Vitamin A is not indestructible, however, because fresh fruits and vegetables rich in vitamin A lose some of their vitamin value when exposed to air for months of storage.

Processed vegetables always lose some of their vitamin value. It is believed that green vegetables lose as much as 20 percent and yellow vegetables maybe a third. The process of drying such foods by exposing them to the air may also cause a significant loss of vitamin A.

TOO MUCH VITAMIN A   Hypervitaminosis A expresses a condition in which the body has taken in and stored too much vitamin A. Toxic signs of vitamin A are peeling and dry skin, headaches, dizziness, nausea, and apathy. In children the symptoms may be vomiting or drowsiness. Those taking moderately large amounts over a long period may notice breaks in the skin at the corners of their mouth or some hair loss.

Since vitamin A is a fat-soluble vitamin stored in body fat, it is usually necessary to consume it only in minute amounts, as found in a multipurpose daily vitamin capsule. For example, a week's supply of vitamin A for most healthy adults is contained in only 2 ounces of beef liver (not chicken liver) or two cups of spinach.

The problem of hypervitaminosis A develops when someone accumulates a total amount that is too high relative to body weight. In some instances the vitamin may become toxic (poisonous) in the body. Those most vulnerable to excessive vitamin A intake are, understandably, those with a low body weight, such as small children. Daily vitamin A supplements should not exceed 2,500 IU unless under a doctor's supervision. An infant may experience vitamin A toxicity within one to three months if given daily doses of 18,000 IU of vitamin A. Another group subject to toxic side effects of megadoses of vitamin A are teenagers eager to cure their acne. Many teenagers wrongly believe that taking more of the vitamin that promotes healthy skin can remedy their skin problem.

DRUG INTERACTIONS   If you are prescribed Colestipol Hydrochloride (Colestid) or Cholestyramine (Questran), two drugs designed to lower your cholesterol count, ask your doctor about the need for vitamin A supplements. People who take Colestid and Questran frequently require supplements of 2,000 to 5,000 IU of vitamin A. (Nutritionists also advise that they take 10 to 15 IU of vitamin E and 200 to 800 IU of vitamin D.)

If you are taking a stool softener on a regular basis (for example, Dioctyl Sodium Sulfosuccinate), the drug may be the cause of a vitamin A deficiency because it inhibits fat absorption. This drug, and others like it, should be accompanied by a daily vitamin supplement containing 500 to 1,000 IU of vitamin A per day. (Nutritionists also recommend a daily supplement of 400 to 800 IU of vitamin D.) No drug, laxatives included, should be taken regularly except under a doctor's supervision.

Mineral oil laxatives (Agoral, Ligui-Doss, Milk of Magnesia-Mineral Oil Emulsion, Milkinol, Whirl-Sol) can interfere with the absorption of vitamin A, and long-term use of many types of antacid drugs can cause a mild deficiency of vitamin A.

Sucralfate (Carafate), a drug taken orally for the treatment of duodenal ulcers and other disorders, will inhibit the absorption of vitamin A if taken over time. It is recommended that you take a vitamin supplement of 2,000 to 5,000 IU of vitamin A while taking this drug. (Nutritionists also advise 10 to 15 IU of vitamin E and 200 to 800 IU of vitamin D.)

SPECIAL ADVICE Many people take megadoses of vitamin E for a variety of speculated and unproven reasons that range from hair loss prevention to enhancement of sexual performance. This practice is unwise, and its risks are compounded by the fact that, while RDA levels of vitamin E aids in the absorption of vitamin A, in megadoses it can actually cause vitamin A stores in the body to be depleted.

VITAMIN D

DESCRIPTION
Vitamin D is important to our health for several reasons. Its primary job is to regulate the metabolism of our dietary calcium and phosphate. Without this vitamin we would not be able to utilize properly the calcium and phosphate to form strong teeth and bones. Our kidneys depend on this vitamin, and it is also instrumental in a smooth-functioning nervous system.

FOOD SOURCES
Excellent Source: fortified foods (for example, milk), fish-liver oils, fatty fish (for example, boiled herring)
Good Source: canned salmon, cream, sardines, tuna, calf's liver, cooked eggs, and cheese

HIGH-RISK GROUPS FOR POSSIBLE DEFICIENCY
- women after menopause
- the elderly
- alchoholics
- people suffering from wasting diseases or severe burns
- people recovering from gastrointestinal surgery
- pregnant or breast-feeding women
- users of Phenytoin (Dilantin), an anti-epileptic drug
- heavy users of Dioctyl Sodium Sulfosuccinate, a drug to soften the stool
- heavy users of Fenfluramine Hydrochloride, a drug to suppress the appetite
- heavy users of Colestipol Hydrochloride (Colestid), a drug that lowers blood cholesterol and triglyceride levels
- users of Doriden, an anti-anxiety drug
- heavy users of mineral oils as a laxative
- long-term use of cathartic laxatives, especially Diphenylmethane cathartics

RECOMMENDED DOSAGE

GROUP	MCG*	GROUP	MCG*
Pregnant women	10	Adult women 19–23	7.5
Lactating women	10	Adult men 11–18	10
Children 1–10	10	19–23	7.5
Adult women 11–18	10	Adults over 23	5

*(Note: 10 mcg = 400 IU)

UPPER LIMITS FOR REGULAR DIETARY SUPPLEMENT USE

Children under 4 years of age: 400 IU
Adults and children 4 or more years of age: 400 IU
Pregnant or lactating women: 400 IU

BENEFITS

TREATMENT OF DEFICIENCY SYMPTOMS
- muscle weakness
- pain in the ribs, spine, and legs
- listlessness
- bone malformation
- osteomalacia

OTHER BENEFITS
- strengthens bones and teeth
- increases blood calcium levels evident in kidney disease
- reduces symptoms of postoperative muscle contractions
- increases calcium and phosphorus absorption

UNPROVEN BENEFITS (UNRELATED TO DEFICIENCY SYMPTOMS)

- prevents herpes
- treats heredity diseases that block fat absorption
- acts as an anti-aging nutrient
- prevents arthritis
- prevents colon cancer

TOXIC SYMPTOMS

High blood pressure, irregular heartbeat, kidney damage, loss of appetite or unexplained weight loss, diarrhea, vomiting, increased thirst, nausea.

DISCOVERY   The story of vitamin D is tied to the story of rickets. Rickets, which is a malformation of the bones due to a deficiency of lime salts (primarily calcium and phosphorus), has been known since 500 B.C. Through the centuries surgeons were able to demonstrate that there was an observable variation in the thickness and quality of human bones by examining the skulls of soldiers slain in battle. (Despite the relative size of a man, it was thought that in normally healthy men the thickness of the human skull was the same.)

In the middle of the seventeenth century the malformation of bones, deformed spines and bowed legs, was known as the *English disease*. In fact, it was an English physician, Francis Glisson, who named the condition *rickets*. (The etymology of the word *rickets* is not clear, but Glisson said he coined it from the Greek word *rachis* which means spinal column. Rickets can cause a softening of the bones of the spinal column.)

During the seventeenth and eighteenth centuries, investigators began to associate the poor hygiene and lack of sunshine and exercise among the London slum children with this deforming disease. In 1824 biochemists were able to prove that cod-liver oil, at that time one of the most widely used foods in folk medicine, was actually an effective treatment for rickets; about seventy years later scientists were able to confirm that the ultraviolet rays of direct sunlight were a cure for rickets. (Anthropologists have speculated that sun worship in primitive societies may have grown out of a similar observation.)

It was another Englishman, Edward Mellanby, who in 1918 provided the first experiment that established rickets as a disease caused by a deficient diet. He was also able to show that cod-liver oil could prevent and cure the disease in puppies. But it was Elmer McCollum in 1922 who identified the curing property in cod-liver oil as being a second fat-soluble vitamin, and it was named vitamin D. McCollum and his associates eventually established that calcium and phosphorus required the presence of vitamin D for proper absorption, and without the vitamin, bones would become weak and soft.

Eventually, when vitamin D was synthesized in a laboratory, it was learned that it was, in fact, a complex of vitamins. Of interest to us are two: vitamins D2 and D3, both of which are effective in human nutrition. Vitamin D2 is found in yeast and fungi, and vitamin D3 occurs naturally in fish oils, egg yolk, and milk. The human skin contains an organic provitamin called a sterol, and when it comes into contact with the ultraviolet rays of sunlight, it is converted into vitamin D3. When this vitamin is formed in or on the skin, it is absorbed into the blood and carried to all parts of the body. For purposes of discussion, however, all these vitamins will be referred to as vitamin D.

The ability to synthesize vitamin D, or any vitamin for that matter, made it possible to add the vitamin to foods poor in it. (In the case of vitamin D, this is critically important because it is not found in abundance in most foods.) Since growing children are in critical need of vitamin D for their growing bones (they need almost twice as much as adults), the first food to be fortified with vitamin D was milk.

Another benefit of this new source of vitamin D was that it could be added inexpensively to animal feed. Fortified animal feed made it possible to raise farm animals indoors (no sunshine) year-round and dramatically lowered the cost of eggs, milk, and meat production in this country. If it weren't for the synthetic vitamin D in fortified pet foods, we couldn't raise our household pets indoors without running the risk of their getting rickets.

ROLE   As studies in rickets revealed, vitamin D is very important in forming strong bones. Specifically, the vitamin is necessary for the formation of a protein in the intestine that is responsible for carrying calcium into the body. Indirectly, vitamin D makes it possible for us to form and maintain healthy strong bones through a process called mineralization. Vitamin D is also important to a healthy heart and to a healthy nervous system because calcium, which is dependent upon the vitamin for proper absorption, is critical for their proper functioning.

PROBLEMS OF TOO LITTLE VITAMIN D   The deficiency disease of vitamin D is rickets. In the absence of sufficient amounts of vitamin D, the minerals of calcium and phosphorus will not deposit in the bones in adequate quantities. Without proper mineralization, the bones grow soft and weak. Bones that become weak will bend under the weight of the body, which accounts for the bowed legs, knock-knees, sunken chest, and narrow pelvis of some children with rickets. None of these disfigurements are life-threatening, but they can cause problems in later life. A sunken chest, for example, can be a further complication for someone with a lung disease, such as asthma, and a narrow pelvis may make child-bearing difficult for some women.

WHO IS AT RISK?   A vitamin D deficiency is seen most dramatically in children because it adversely affects their skeletal frame and posture. The growing bones of children depend on the proper utilization of dietary calcium and phosphorus, and vitamin D is absolutely indispensable in the process.

Most children in this country are reasonably well protected from any vitamin D deficiency because it is now a routine supplement in all commercial infant formulas. Breast-fed infants routinely are given 400 IU of vitamin D because the level of vitamin D in the mother's milk is quite low. It is believed that the vitamin does not get passed on in the mother's breast milk to any significant degree.

Although vitamin D deficiency is not common in adults, it does occur occasionally during pregnancy. The profile of someone at risk would be a woman who has had many pregnancies, whose diet is deficient, and who possibly has had very little exposure to the sun (someone who has been housebound during most of her pregnancy).

As with all the fat-soluble vitamins, people who have suffered severe burns, are recovering from gastrointestinal surgery, or are suffering from a wasting disease may require significantly more vitamin D than is provided in their daily diet.

STRATEGIES

FOODS SOURCES We should look beyond our diet for vitamin D because there is precious little of it in plant and animal foods. In fact, it is the most scarce of all the vitamins. Thanks to sunlight, though, we have an easily accessible source of vitamin D, and despite its scarcity, there are some foods we can add to our diet that are rich in the vitamin: fatty fish and the organs of animals (calf's liver).

The vitamin D value in any animal food will vary according to the diet of the animal and how much it was exposed to sunlight. You'll note on the table for Vitamin D-Rich Foods (see page 264) that it is a relatively brief list, and it does not include any vegetables, fruits, or grain because they have little or no vitamin D activity.

SPECIAL ADVICE All homogenized, skim, and evaporated milk sold in this country is fortified by 400 IU of vitamin D per liquid quart, which is the recommended daily allowance set by the government.

TOO MUCH VITAMIN D Fat-soluble vitamins, such as vitamin D are stored in body fat, primarily in the liver, so it is not essential to consume them daily except in minute amounts. For healthy adults there is no evidence that any benefits are added if more of the vitamin is taken than is required. It may be impossible to say precisely what the exact human requirements for vitamin D are, but the Food and Nutrition Board believes that 400 IU of vitamin D daily from birth to the age of twenty-two is sufficient to meet most needs. Most healthy adults need only 200 IU unless they are pregnant or lactating, suffering from a disease, or taking medication that interferes with the vitamin. (Pregnant or lactating women should take 400 IU per day.)

As for what is too much, there is evidence that infants with intakes as low as 1,800 to 3,000 IU per day can become toxic. These quantities have produced abnormally high calcium blood levels—hypercalcemia—resulting in diarrhea and poor growth performance. Children receiving megadoses of 20,000 IU and adults taking as much as 75,000 IU have experienced serious toxic problems. In children it has resulted in retarded growth; in adults, irreversible kidney damage. Some other potential risks of megadoses are hearing loss, high blood pressure, increased cholesterol levels, nausea, and loss of appetite. Some people have had symptoms of an irregular heartbeat and kidney damage.

In summary, unused fat-soluble vitamin D will remain in the body and, over time, if the excess continues to accumulate, will become toxic to the body. Clearly, megadoses of vitamin D are risky business.

DRUG INTERACTIONS   If you are prescribed Colestipol Hydrochloride (Colestid) or Cholestyramine (Questran), two drugs designed to lower your cholesterol count, ask your doctor about the need for vitamin D supplements. People who take Colestid and Questran over time frequently require supplements of 200 to 800 IU of vitamin D.

Phenytoin (Dilantin), an anti-epileptic drug, can accelerate the metabolism of vitamin D and jeopardize its proper utilization in your liver. Another drug, Phenobarbital, which is a strong sedative, can also create a mild vitamin D deficiency. In both of these instances, nutritionists may recommend taking 400 to 800 IU of vitamin D daily while on these medications.

Fenfluramine Hydrochloride (Pondimin) is an appetite suppressant used in the treatment of obesity. It is the most effective suppressant available, but over time it could impair absorption of fats and fat-soluble vitamins. Since the drug is additive, it should not be prescribed for long periods, thereby also reducing the threat of a vitamin deficiency.

Primidone (Mysoline), an anti-epileptic drug that, among other things, increases the destruction of vitamin D, and Sucralfate (Carafate), a drug taken orally for the treatment of duodenal ulcers, also inhibit the absorption of vitamin D if taken over time.

If you are using a stool softener on a regular basis (for example, Dioctyl Sodium Sulfosuccinate), the drug may be the cause of a vitamin D deficiency because it inhibits fat absorption. Another category of laxatives called cathartics, such as Diphenylmethane Cathartic, can also create a malabsorption of vitamin D. Because mineral oil is largely indigestible, mineral oil laxatives (Agoral, Ligui-Doss, Milk of Magnesia-Mineral Oil Emulsion, Milkinol, Whirl-Sol) will capture vitamin D and prevent it from being absorbed.

If these drugs are taken frequently, it is advised that you take a daily supplement of 400 to 800 IU of vitamin D.

VITAMIN E

DESCRIPTION

Vitamin E is thought to have a broad range of functions in maintaining our physical and emotional health. It is central to the formation of red blood cells, muscles, and other tissues in the body. It is a substance that opposes oxidation, which means it inhibits many of the destructive reactions promoted by oxygen. As an antioxidant, the vitamin is able to protect the vitamin A and vital fatty acids of our body from destruction. Studies involving gross deficiencies of vitamin A indicate that vitamin E is necessary for a healthy functioning nervous system, too. Although still speculated, there is some evidence that the vitamin may have some significant healing properties.

FOOD SOURCES

Excellent Sources: dry soy beans, wheat germ oil, soybean oil, cottonseed oil, corn oil, margarine (tub corn oil), and dry lima beans
Good Sources: sunflower seeds, walnuts, pecans, peanuts (dry roasted), wheat germ (cereal), and fresh raw spinach

HIGH-RISK GROUPS FOR POSSIBLE DEFICIENCY

- people who abuse alcohol and other drugs
- people recovering from gastrointestinal surgery or severe burns
- the elderly
- people suffering from a wasting disease
- heavy users of Colestipol Hydrochloride (Colestid) or Cholestyramine (Questran), two drugs that lower blood cholesterol and triglyceride levels
- heavy users of antacids

RECOMMENDED DOSAGE

GROUP	MG	GROUP	MG
Pregnant women	10	Children 11–15	8
Lactating women	11	15–18	10
Children 1–10	5–7	Adults	10

UPPER LIMITS FOR REGULAR DIETARY SUPPLEMENT USE

Children under 4 years of age: 15 mg
Adults and children 4 or more years of age: 45 mg
Pregnant or lactating women: 60 mg

BENEFITS

TREATING DEFICIENCY SYMPTOMS

- weakness
- irritability
- listlessness
- diarrhea
- poor skin condition

OTHER POSSIBLE BENEFITS

- treats problems associated with oxidation in the body
- anti-blood-clotting agent
- protects vitamin A
- aids red blood cell production

UNPROVEN BENEFITS (UNRELATED TO DEFICIENCY SYMPTOMS)

- improves sexual performance
- treats infertility
- reduces the effects of scars
- treats acne
- improves circulation in legs and feet
- treats burns by direct application to the skin
- lowers blood pressure
- treats rheumatism
- treats cystitis
- treats colitis

TOXIC SYMPTOMS

Blurred vision, diarrhea, headaches, dizziness, flu-like symptoms, breast enlargement in males and females, excessive fatigue, loss of appetite, nausea, and persistent flatulence.

DISCOVERY   In 1922 two chemists at the University of California, Dr. Herbert Evans and Dr. Katherine Bishop, discovered the third fat-soluble substance (the first two were vitamins A and D). The fertility of rats raised on a diet deficient in certain foods declined in the first generation, and they became sterile in the second generation. When the rats were given a diet of lettuce, yeast, and other foods, their condition was completely reversed. Two years later the name vitamin E was given to this newest of fat-soluble vitamins.

In 1936 Dr. Evans isolated a crystalline form of vitamin E from wheat germ oil and named it *tocopherol,* from the Greek words *tokos* (birth) and *pherein* (to carry). Generally, *tocopherol* is translated as "to bear offspring."

In 1938 biochemists determined that vitamin E was naturally available in four different forms, called alpha, beta, gamma, and delta-tocopherols.

ROLE   Vitamin E is found in all the tissues of the body. The adrenal and pituitary glands show high concentrations, but the vitamin is stored primarily in the fatty and muscle tissues of the body. Vitamin E's task is to protect other compounds, such as fatty acids and vitamin A, from destruction. These fat-containing substances are destroyed by oxygen because the oxygen molecule breaks down fat, decomposes it, and subsequently makes the fat rancid. As a powerful antioxidant, vitamin E draws off the oxygen and prevents the fatty tissue from becoming rancid. In much the same way, the vitamin protects the supply of the fat-soluble vitamin A in the body. This protection is especially important for someone whose intake or store of vitamin A is poor.

As an antioxidant, vitamin E also helps protect the red blood cells from oxidizing agents, and it probably plays a very positive role in making most, if not all, of our body membranes less fragile and open to destruction.

PROBLEMS OF TOO LITTLE VITAMIN E   Vitamin E is widely available in our diet, which explains the virtual non-existence of a naturally occurring deficiency in the United States. Another reason most of us will never experience a vitamin E deficiency is that our storage capacity is very extensive. Clinical studies designed to produce a deficiency have found it necessary to require patients to eat a three-year diet virtually free of vitamin E to produce significant deficiency symptoms. Finally, we use very little of it at any one time.

If the preservation of fat and fatty acids depends on an appropriate amount of vitamin E, then an increase in fats and fatty acids calls for an increase in the vitamin. By way of example, the more you increase your intake of linoleic acid or other polyunsaturated fatty acids, the more you concurrently increase your requirement for vitamin E.

WHO IS AT RISK   The deficiencies that have occurred have been among adults whose diets were consistently low in vitamin E and high in polyunsaturated fatty acids. Newborn infants, especially premature babies, occasionally need supplemental E because of a poor transfer of the vitamin from the mother. Nursing does not pose a threat of a vitamin deficiency because, unlike vitamin A, a mother's milk is generally a good source of vitamin E. Cow's milk, on the other hand, is a relatively poor source of vitamin E. Consequently, commercial baby formulas are fortified with vitamin E, but some people still believe that the iron in these formulas oxidizes the vitamin E, reducing the amount available for the infant.

Another group at risk of a vitamin E deficiency are those who have a problem absorbing fats and oils, such as those with cystic fibrosis, cirrhosis of the liver, obstructive jaundice, or hyperthyroidism. People who have suffered severe burns, are recovering from gastrointestinal surgery, or are suffering from a wasting disease may have absorption problems that can adversely affect their vitamin E level.

STRATEGIES

FOOD SOURCES   Some of the better natural sources of vitamin E are dry lima beans and dry soy beans. Nuts (for example, almonds and peanuts) and seeds (for example, sunflower seeds) are relatively good sources as well. Among cereals, wheat germ is the outstanding choice, but oatmeal and cornmeal are also moderate to good sources of vitamin E. The yolk of a raw egg is a source, but if it is fried (as opposed to a quick soft boiling in the shell), it may lose some of its vitamin value. As you will note on the food table for vitamin E (see page 264), there are no fruits listed; this is because they contain very little vitamin E. For much the same reason, fish does not make the list, with the exception of the oil from codfish.

FOOD PREPARATION   Fish oils (for example, cod-liver oil), plant oils (for example, soybean oil), and the oils drawn from nuts provide the richest available food source of vitamin E. These oils are light yellow and viscous, and are insoluble in water, and are not easily destroyed by normal cooking temperatures. However, vitamin E can be destroyed by ultraviolet light and oxygen, and some vitamin loss occurs in processed foods; as much as 80 percent may be lost in converting whole wheat to white bread. Unlike most vitamins, the vitamin E in vegetables (for example, spinach and asparagus) can be lost if the food is frozen.

Because "fast foods" or "convenience foods" are usually highly processed, they contribute very little vitamin E to our diet. There are a number of prepared food products on the market, however, that can be fairly reliable sources of vitamin E, depending upon the oils used. Check the labels of preparations, such as salad dressings and margarines, to see if they have used oils rich in vitamin E, such as corn oil. The best bet is a cold-pressed oil, such as olive oil, whose vitamin E value is virtually intact because it has not been processed or is only marginally refined. They can be found in the health food section of your market and in a good food specialty shop. We get about two-thirds of our vitamin E intake through our use of these oils and commercial preparations in our diets; the balance comes primarily from whole grains, beans, vegetables, and beef liver.

TOO MUCH VITAMIN E   There is virtually no risk of ever getting too much vitamin E in your regular diet through food sources. Megadoses of vitamin E supplements can cause a problem, however. In most cases vitamin supplements should be taken only if you cannot get enough vitamin E in your diet since a balanced diet should provide all that a healthy person needs.

Admittedly, there may be an occasion when supplements are necessary, but large doses of the vitamin should not be taken over a long period without a doctor's supervision or a sound medical reason. If you suffer from a known deficiency or a disease that you believe requires higher amounts of vitamin E than is recommended by the RDA, consult your doctor before treating the problem with a program of vitamin E therapy. And don't forget that the total amount of vitamins ingested each day includes what you get from the foods you eat and what you take as supplements.

If you use vitamin E supplements, understand that the activity or potency of synthetic vitamin E may be less than the vitamin in its natural form. Animal studies indicate that synthetic vitamin E is far less active (in some cases almost two-thirds) and therefore less effective compared with vitamin E in its natural form. This is no justification to consume more of the vitamin in its synthetic form as compensation for the difference. Look to your diet for help.

SPECIAL ADVICE   Since synthetic and natural vitamin E may not have the same value, how can we tell on a label which is which? If it's a synthetic vitamin E, the listing of the ingredient will begin with *dl* or end with *yl* (for example, *dl'alpha-tocopheryl*). If the vitamin is present in its natural form and is listed by its proper name, it will begin with a *d*, such as *d'alpha-tocopherol*. Other natural forms are beta, gamma, and delta-tocopherol, or mixed tocopherol. Finally, if listed as "vitamin E," it is a natural and synthetic mixture.

DRUG INTERACTIONS   If your doctor has prescribed Colestipol Hydrochloride (Colestid) or Cholestyramine (Questran), two drugs designed to lower your cholesterol count, ask the doctor about the need for vitamin E supplements. People who take Colestid and Questran over time frequently require supplements of 10 to 15 IU of vitamin E.

Anyone taking drugs that thin the blood, such as Dicumarol or Warfarin (Coumadin, Panwarfin, Warfarin Sodium), must be aware that these drugs are hostile to vitamin E and can cause a deficiency of the vitamin.

Taken over time, Sucralfate (Carafate), a drug taken orally for a variety of disorders including the treatment of duodenal ulcers, will inhibit the absorption of vitamin E.

Iron supplements, which are needed to raise red blood cell production, are usually prescribed in the case of iron deficiency anemia. If taken in amounts that exceed the RDA allowances, the iron supplement can destroy vitamin E stores in the body. The long-term use of many types of antacid preparations can decrease vitamin E absorption that could result in a mild deficiency as well. Mineral oil laxatives (Agoral, Ligui-Doss, Milk of Magnesia-Mineral Oil Emulsion, Milkinol, Whirl-Sol), can also interfere with the absorption of vitamin E.

VITAMIN K

DESCRIPTION

The fourth fat-soluble vitamin is vitamin K. As you should assume by its designated letter, it was the last vitamin of this fat-soluble category to be discovered and named. Its only known function is the formation in the liver of a protein called prothrombin, which is necessary for coagulation, or clotting, of the blood. It is a most important function since it is routinely given to newborn infants to prevent bleeding.

FOOD SOURCES

Excellent Sources: alfalfa, turnip greens, cooked broccoli, beef liver, cooked spinach
Good Sources: asparagus, cabbage, cheese, rolled oats, watercress, egg yolks, soybean oil, cauliflower, and tomatoes

HIGH-RISK GROUPS FOR POSSIBLE DEFICIENCY

- premature newborns
- people with cancer
- people recovering from gastrointestinal surgery or severe burns
- heavy users of antacids
- heavy users of mineral oils or a drug called Sucralfate that is used to treat ulcers
- heavy users of Colestipol Hydrochloride (Colestid) or Cholestyramine (Questran), two drugs that lower blood cholesterol and triglyceride levels
- people who are taking antibiotics
- people who are taking anticoagulants such as Warfarin (Coumadin, Panwarfin, and Warafin Sodium)
- chronic users of aspirin

RECOMMENDED DOSAGE

GROUP	IU	GROUP	IU
Pregnant women	70–140	Children 4–6	20–40
Lactating women	70–140	7–10	30–60
Infants 0–.6	12	11–18	50–100
.6–1	10–20	Adults	70–140
Children 1–3	15–30		

UPPER LIMITS FOR REGULAR DIETARY SUPPLEMENT USE

Children under 4 years of age: Not established
Adults and children 4 or more years of age: Not established
Pregnant or lactating women: Not established

BENEFITS

TREATING DEFICIENCY SYMPTOMS

INFANTS
- feeding problems
- vomiting blood
- failure to grow normally

ADULTS
- abnormal nosebleeds
- blood in the urine
- spontaneous bruises (black-and-blue marks)
- prolonged clotting time (determined through test results)
- internal hemorrhage (gross deficiency)

OTHER POSSIBLE BENEFITS
- treats bleeding problems in those taking anticoagulant medicines

UNPROVEN BENEFITS (UNRELATED TO DEFICIENCY SYMPTOMS)

- protects against cancer-causing agents
- treats celiac disease
- treats cystic fibrosis
- prevents cerebral palsy

TOXIC SYMPTOMS

From prescribed or synthetic vitamin K preparations only: Flushing of the face and, in rare cases, liver damage.

DISCOVERY   Vitamin K was discovered in 1935 by a Danish biochemist, Dr. Carl Dam, well-known at that time for his work on how chicken hens synthesized cholesterol. Dr. Dam observed that none of the known vitamins would clear up the small hemorrhages the chicks developed when fed a synthetic diet. He concluded that a vitamin must exist in some foods that assisted coagulation, and he proposed that it be called *koagulation vitamin* (German spelling), from which the name vitamin K evolved. Dr. Dam and Dr. Edward Doisy, an American biochemist in St. Louis who determined the chemical structure of the vitamin in 1939, shared the Nobel Prize in 1943 for their work.

DIFFERENT VITAMIN KS   Vitamin K appears in several different forms. Primarily, vitamins K1 and K2 are two natural forms. Vitamin K1 is found in plants, especially green leafy plants; vitamin K2 is the form that is synthesized by bacteria in our intestinal tract. Another form, sometimes referred to as vitamin K3, is the vitamin in its synthetic form. For our discussion, however, we will refer to them all as vitamin K.

ROLE   Vitamin K, unlike its fellow fat-soluble vitamins, is produced in the intestine of our body by intestinal bacteria. Two American scientists in 1919 established that more than half of the newborns at that time may have had unknown hemorrhages due to undeveloped intestinal bacteria.

The significance of vitamin production by the intestinal bacteria was not easily accepted by many doctors. Some found it difficult to believe that the avowed enemy of mankind could ever serve as a friend. Even in the late 1940s, prominent doctors with their reputations very much at stake held out against embracing the theory that bacteria could produce vitamins. As unlikely as this dispute may seem, a full understanding of the blood-clotting mechanism is still unknown today.

Vitamin K is synthesized in our small intestine and absorbed through the intestinal wall into the body with the help of body fats and bile produced in the liver. Along with the other fat-soluble vitamins, it is stored in the liver where the vitamin produces the protein enzyme *prothrombin*. This protein is then converted to its active form—*thrombin*— and used to produce yet another protein called *fibrin*, the substance that is the basis for a blood clot.

TOO LITTLE VITAMIN K   A naturally occurring vitamin K deficiency is unlikely because, in addition to the synthesis of the vitamin in the body, our average daily diet provides two to three times the amount needed.

WHO IS AT RISK   Deficiencies of vitamin K do occur, especially in premature infants because the infant is born with low values of plasma-clotting factors and lacks the intestinal flora or bacteria to synthesize or produce adequate levels of vitamin K. Vitamin K is critical to the production of prothrombin and other clotting factors, and therefore the infant is usually given a small dose of vitamin K by injection.

Because anticoagulants interfere with the synthesis of vitamin K, babies born to mothers taking these drugs are often deficient. Expectant mothers who are prescribed this type of drug during their pregnancy are given additional vitamin K during the last month in routine prenatal care to help raise the newborn's level of vitamin K. It is also the practice to add vitamin K supplements to the newborn's formula.

Deficiencies have occurred in babies receiving drugs for diarrhea or intestinal infections. Both the drug and the disorders could block the absorption of the vitamin to create a vitamin deficiency. It is not a major problem to treat the deficiency, however, since a normal infant's daily requirement is approximately 15 micrograms, the amount present in about a quart of human milk. (Cow's milk is somewhat richer in vitamin K than human milk.)

When a vitamin K deficiency occurs in adults, it is usually the result of medication or a disease that negatively affects the absorption or the production of the vitamin in the intestine. In fact, any drug that destroys the intestinal bacterial flora required to produce vitamin K will affect vitamin K production.

Anyone who suffers from chronic diarrhea or ulcerative colitis may develop a deficiency because these conditions interfere with vitamin K absorption. Disorders that affect the flow of bile salts or its production, such as obstructive jaundice (bile ducts are blocked) or liver disease (where bile salts are produced), can produce a vitamin K deficiency because bile salts are necessary for absorption of the vitamin.

Vitamin K deficiencies have appeared in animals as well as humans—sometimes for the same reasons. Vitamin K deficiencies were at one time commonplace in poultry flocks, for example, because of the widespread use of sulfur drugs in disease prevention. Humans develop a similar deficiency with certain drug use. (See Drug Interactions, page 77). It was only after synthetic forms of the vitamin were developed and introduced into the diet of the animal, along with dried alfalfa (one of the richest sources of vitamin K), that the problems vanished.

TOO MUCH VITAMIN K   Vitamin K in its natural form is not known to become toxic even when consumed in relatively large amounts. On the other hand, a synthetic form of the vitamin called menadione (once known as vitamin K3) has been associated with toxic symptoms. In relatively low amounts it has produced jaundice in infants, and it has produced some liver damage in adults. Consequently, the FDA does not allow menadione in any food supplements or vitamin pills. In fact, this therapeutic form of the vitamin K can be purchased only through a doctor's prescription.

STRATEGIES

FOOD SOURCES   Because a healthy intestinal tract produces vitamin K, our average American diet usually provides adequate amounts. Sources include all the green leafy vegetables (for example, lettuce, cabbage, turnip greens, and spinach), broccoli, egg yolks, soybean oil, liver, cauliflower, and tomatoes.

There are many foods that contain little or no vitamin K; for example, it is virtually nonexistent in most fruits, cereals, yellow vegetables, meats, and highly refined foods. In the foods containing vitamin K, it is not often evenly distributed; in green vegetables, for example: The innermost leaves of a head of cabbage contain probably one-fourth as much as the outer leaves.

In addition to these sources of vitamin K, fermented dairy products such as yogurt and buttermilk are important because they will promote growth of the bacterial flora that is central to the synthesis of the vitamin.

FOOD PREPARATION Vitamin K is stable in heat, air, and moisture. Since it is insoluble in water, very little of the vitamin is destroyed in cooking. Like vitamin E, however, it can be destroyed if exposed to sunlight or if it is cooked for long periods in fat.

On balance, none of the vitamin K is lost in cooking except for the little that may be destroyed if the food is cooked in hot fat. It is estimated that a balanced diet contains 300 to 500 micrograms of vitamin K per day, which is far more than is needed.

DRUG INTERACTIONS Anyone taking drugs that thin the blood, such as Dicumarol or Warfarin (Coumadin, Panwarfin, Warafin Sodium), must be aware that these drugs are hostile to vitamin K and can cause a possible deficiency. Common sense tells us that these drugs are all the more likely to cause such a deficiency if the person taking the drug has an abnormally low intake of dietary vitamin K.

Colestipol Hydrochloride (Colestid) and Cholestyramine (Questran), two drugs designed to lower the cholesterol count, impair vitamin K absorption. Over time, Sucralfate (Carafate), a drug taken orally for the treatment of duodenal ulcers, can also inhibit its absorption.

Primidone (Mysoline), an anti-epileptic drug, destroys vitamin K at a rapid rate, which means it can produce a vitamin K deficiency. Your doctor may prescribe a vitamin K supplement of 100 micrograms per day while taking the drug. During this time vitamin E supplements should not be taken because they impair the absorption of vitamin K.

Many antibiotic drugs, such as Kanamycin (Kantrex), suppress the growth of intestinal bacteria. Deficiencies of vitamin K can occur if this type of drug is used over several weeks. Although it is rather rare, people who abuse aspirin, with a daily consumption of 30 milligrams or more, develop a need for vitamin K, too.

Mineral oil laxatives (Agoral, Ligui-Doss, Milk of Magnesia-Mineral Oil Emulsion, Milkinol, Whirl-Sol) interfere with the absorption of vitamin K, and any long-term use of antacids can bring about a mild deficiency in vitamin K.

In all of these instances of a potential vitamin K deficiency, it is advised that you first increase your intake of foods rich in vitamin K. Only if you are experiencing symptoms of a vitamin K deficiency should you take vitamin K supplements, and then the daily dosage should not exceed 100 micrograms per day without the supervision of a physician.

VITAMIN C

DESCRIPTION

The principal function of vitamin C is to maintain collagen, a protein necessary in the formation of connective tissue in skin, ligaments, and bones. It strengthens the dentin (the main tissue) in teeth and is important in helping to prevent plaque formation on teeth. It also plays a role in healing wounds and burns because it facilitates the formation of connective tissue in the scar. It aids in the formation of red blood cells, strengthens blood vessels, and helps prevent hemorrhaging. It fights bacterial infections, aids iron absorption, and protects vitamins A and E from degrading.

FOOD SOURCES

Excellent Sources: red peppers, orange juice, lemon juice, collards, broccoli, brussels sprouts, green peppers, and peaches

Good Sources: grapefruit juice, cranberry juice, lime juice, raw parsley, kale, asparagus, and spinach

HIGH-RISK GROUPS FOR POSSIBLE DEFICIENCY

- people recovering from gastrointestinal surgery or severe burns
- alcoholics and alcoholics being treated with the drug Paraldehyde
- pregnant or breast-feeding women
- people over the age of 55
- people on low-calorie diets
- people suffering from a chronic wasting disease or acute fevers
- chronic users of aspirin
- people using Tetracycline, an antibiotic drug
- people taking corticosteroids, which are drugs to treat inflammation
- people taking barbiturates
- women taking oral contraceptives
- heavy cigarette smokers

RECOMMENDED DOSAGE

GROUP	MG	GROUP	MG
Pregnant women	80	Children 7–10	45
Lactating women	100	11–18	50
Infants 0–.6	35	Adults	60
.6–1	35	Heavy cigarette smokers	100
Children 1–3	45		
4–6	45		

UPPER LIMITS FOR REGULAR DIETARY SUPPLEMENT USE

Children under 4 years of age: 60 mg
Adults and children 4 or more years of age: 90 mg
Pregnant or lactating women: 120 mg

BENEFITS

TREATING DEFICIENCY SYMPTOMS

- urinary tract infections
- scurvy
- bleeding or spongy gums
- abnormal nosebleeds
- anemia
- healing of wounds
- pinpoint bruising
- swollen ankles and wrists

OTHER POSSIBLE BENEFITS

- helps block nitrosamines
- treats iron-deficiency anemia
- used in treatment of broken bones

UNPROVEN BENEFITS (UNRELATED TO DEFICIENCY SYMPTOMS)

- protects against cancer-causing agents
- cures the common cold
- protects against heart attacks
- reduces rectal polyps
- prevents allergies
- heals bedsores
- helps relieve herpes
- reduces cholesterol

TOXIC SYMPTOMS

Flushed face, increased urination, diarrhea, abdominal cramps

DISCOVERY   The story of vitamin C is perhaps the longest in all of nutritional history. Like a number of other vitamins, its discovery is tied to the disease that is caused by its deficiency—scurvy.

Our evidence of scurvy reaches as far back as 1500 B.C. to the city of Thebes. It also appears in the writings of Hippocrates as early as 400 B.C. It was so widespread throughout fifteenth- and sixteenth-century Europe that many thought all diseases were indirectly related to scurvy.

In the late sixteenth century it was also known as the scourge of the seas—with good reason. Sir Richard Hawkins, a British seaman and politician of that time, said that at least ten thousand seamen died of scurvy.

Famous sea voyages were plagued by the disease. Vasco da Gama lost 100 of his 150 men to scurvy in 1497, and Magellan lost nearly half his crew in his circumnavigation in 1520. But perhaps the most dramatic example of the terror of scurvy is the tale of one Lord Anson who left England in 1740 with six ships and a crew of 961. When he returned three and a half years later he brought back only one ship and 190 men; the rest were all lost to scurvy.

Records of the crusaders of the Middle Ages suggest that they believed the pain in their legs and feet and their bleeding gums would be cured by a move to a warmer climate, which meant that fresh fruit and vegetables would be more available.

When the Spaniards first arrived in California they spoke of searching for an herb to cure scurvy. (If only they had sought out the potato, an export from Central and South America to most of Europe, their problem would have been solved since it is a good source of vitamin C.) In the nineteenth century the Mormons migrating west recorded many deaths when they were forced to winter in Nebraska. In fact, throughout history armies all over the world have reported the devastations of scurvy, and the outcome of many siege battles was determined by the number of soldiers, or citizens, lost to scurvy.

The search for a cure for scurvy centers on the work of James Lind, a Scottish physician. After observing that the disease flourished in beseiged towns and on long sea voyages where the diet was limited and monotonous, Lind was convinced that it was caused by a deficient diet. To test his theory, in 1747 he divided sailors afflicted with scurvy into six pairs and fed them six different diets, including the ship's basic diet. Among the different diets he tried oil of vitriol (sulfuric acid) in water, vinegar, extract of ginger, cinnamon, and alcohol. The only sailors that improved were those fed a diet he fashioned from oranges and lemons. Within six days the sailors who were fed his diet were cured of the disease and returned to duty, whereas those on the other diets showed virtually no improvement.

What was revolutionary about this experiment, which Dr. Lind published as the *Treatise on Scurvy,* was not only that it solved the mystery of the dreaded scurvy and provided a cure, but it also held out the possibility that other diseases were caused by a deficient diet. Inexplicably, the British admiralty waited another fifty years before they recognized the benefits of Dr. Lind's findings and mandated that all ships leaving British ports must carry for its crew sufficient lime juice for the entire voyage.

The modern story of vitamin C picks up about 1912 when the scurvy-preventing substance in limes was being referred to as the "scurvy vitamine" or the "antiscorbutim" compound. But the credit for the official discovery of the vitamin concerns a dispute. In 1928 the Hungarian-born scientist Albert Szent-Gyorgyi (St. George) isolated a substance from the adrenal gland that appeared to be much the same as a substance he later obtained from cabbages and oranges. This led him to suspect that the substance we now know as ascorbic acid was a vitamin. (*Ascorbic* means no scurvy.)

Szent-Gyorgyi's substance was called hexuronic acid because it contained six (*hexa* in Latin means six) atoms of carbon. What is important is that even though he knew there was a firm relationship between the two substances, he never bothered to test whether hexuronic acid was, in fact, the same antiscurvy substance extracted from these two foods. Had he carried out the experiment, which was a very simple, routine procedure with test animals, his claims to the discovery of vitamin C would not have been contested.

By this time Charles Glen King, an American biochemist, had already isolated from lemon juice a crystalline substance that proved to have antiscorbutic properties. But he, too, did not experiment with the possible connection between Szent-Gyorgyi's compound and his. Another American scientist, Joseph Svirbely, who knew both King and Szent-Gyorgyi, decided to act on his own suspicions and, with the permission of Szent-Gyorgyi, tested the two substances. He learned that King's crystalline substance and hexuronic acid were identical; both were capable of curing guinea pigs of scurvy.

As a professional courtesy he wrote his former colleague, Charles Glen King, and told him that his crystalline substance was the long-sought vitamin C, which was the same as hexuronic acid. Svirbely also shared the laboratory evidence with Szent-Gyorgyi. The result was that King beat Szent-Gyorgyi into print with this news, by sixteen days, which caused many people to believe that King and Svirbely should have received official credit for the discovery of vitamin C. It was Szent-Gyorgyi, however, who received the Nobel Prize in 1937 for his work on vitamin C. The American press accused him of stealing the prize but, in the judgment of the awards committee, it was Szent-Gyorgyi's pioneering work that was decisive. Besides, it was the view of the Nobel committee that many people had contributed to the discovery of the vitamin, and it was against policy to award a Nobel prize for science to more than three individuals.

ROLE Maybe the best understood function of vitamin C is its role in forming a protein component that acts as a "mortar" in all connective tissue. This mortar, called collagen, is essential in binding together the cells of connective tissue. It also is a component of scar tissue, skin, cartilage, teeth, and bone. The bone matrix, which is one-fifth of the total weight of the bone, is made up of collagen. When vitamin C is lacking, the matrix is impaired and the bone becomes less capable of retaining calcium and phosphorus during calcification. The consequence is that the bone is weakened. If there is a vitamin C deficiency, the cartilage, which is also primarily collagen, may become weakened, resulting in dislocations. During the critical period of teeth formation, a lack of vitamin C may produce a structural weakness that makes the tooth less resistant to decay and breakage in later years. Because of its role in forming scar tissue, some researchers believe vitamin C should be part of any therapy following surgery. In support of that policy is the evidence that suggests skin grafts heal more quickly when vitamin C is present. Whether this means that the patient requires more than the usual intake is still undecided.

Vitamin C has a number of relationships with other nutrients. It aids in the conversion of two amino acids, tyrosine and tryptophan, which lead to the formation of two neurotransmitters, norepinephrine and serotonin, respectively. These neurotransmitters are required to transfer nerve impulses from one cell to another. Vitamin C also aids in the absorption of dietary iron and its transfer into the liver.

Of the growing number of benefits ascribed to vitamin C, it should be said that the vitamin may reduce or mask many symptoms but never actually correct the underlying health problem.

TOO LITTLE VITAMIN C A gross vitamin C deficiency is rare. When it does occur, however, the early symptoms are relatively nonspecific: fatigue, general weakness, shortness of breath, muscle cramps, aching bones and joints, and loss of appetite. A more telling symptom is the pinpoint hemorrhages called *petechiae* (*petecchia* in Italian means skin spot). These hemorrhages will appear when the body's normal store of vitamin C, which is about 1,500 milligrams, declines to about 300 milligrams. In one experiment people who were placed on a severe vitamin C-deficient diet for a month began to exhibit these pinpoint hemorrhages.

WHO IS AT RISK Scurvy, which is the most dramatic and serious sign of a vitamin C deficiency, is seldom seen in this country. When it does occur, referred to as latent scurvy, it usually appears in infants (after the age of six months) and young children. (Rarely do newborns have deficiency symptoms.) To provide adequate protection for the infant who is breast-feeding, it is recommended that the lactating mother take 100 milligrams of vitamin C, which is easily obtained from two servings of citrus fruit juice. One reason for pregnant women to keep their vitamin C intake within prescribed margins is that infants born to mothers who have consumed high intakes during their pregnancy have a "conditioned" need for vitamin C higher than the amount available in breast milk or baby formulas.

The elderly tend to produce less hydrochloric acid, which adversely affects their absorption of iron. Nutritionists recommend that citrus fruits be added to their diet because the citric acid can compensate for the loss of gastric acid and facilitate iron absorption. People on severe low-calorie diets or those who generally have poor eating habits, such as many of the elderly, may be at some risk of deficiency symptoms. Alcoholics sometimes show evidence of a need for vitamin C because of their inadequate diets and because alcohol destroys the vitamin. Heavy smokers are exposed to a loss of vitamin C because tobacco negatively affects the vitamin. (It is not clear whether tobacco decreases its absorption or actually destroys the vitamin.) People who are heavy users of aspirin are also at some risk because aspirin causes the body to retain less of the vitamin. For example, people with arthritis who take twelve or more aspirins daily for the treatment of their disease are likely to see some deficiency signs, such as bleeding gums and easy bruising.

Vitamin C deficiency symptoms are more likely to appear in those whose intake is insufficient during periods of an increased need of the vitamin, such as growth periods for children, long periods of physiological stress, and when fever is present. Symptoms in young children are signs of irritability and poor growth, restlessness or weakness, and swollen joints. The symptoms in older children and adults are a lack of energy or endurance, small hemorrhages under the skin (petechiae), and gums that are spongy or bleed easily.

NOTE The amount of vitamin C in human milk is higher than that in cow's milk primarily because much of the vitamin is destroyed in the heat processing. Therefore, cow's milk cannot meet the vitamin C needs of the infant after the first two weeks. Most baby formulas have enough vitamin C added to take care of any losses during sterilization. (It is recommended that bottle-fed infants receive a supplement of 35 milligrams and premature infants receive double that amount.) Fruit juices other than citrus juices will not provide enough vitamin C for the infant.

Furthermore, the practice of giving newborn infants orange juice as a source of vitamin C was dropped when it was discovered that the oil from the orange rind caused allergic reactions. Newborns are now given synthetic vitamin C for the first few months, after which fruit juice appears to be quite safe.

TOO MUCH VITAMIN C   Vitamin C is water soluble, and it is not stored in significant quantities in the body. Consequently, many people believe there is no danger in taking megadoses of the vitamin (at least ten times the amount recommended) because the unused amounts will be passed out in the urine. It is true that vitamin C is nontoxic but it is also a chemical, and at excessively high levels toxic symptoms can develop. People who have consumed more than 1,000 milligrams per day have absorbed excessive iron and excreted high levels of uric acid in their urine (a sign of possible gout). The fact is that the body can store only about 250 milligrams. If daily intakes exceed 250 to 300 milligrams, the body will become saturated, not absorb the extra amounts, and excrete them.

POSSIBLE BENEFITS TO INCREASED DOSES OF VITAMIN C Much has been said and written about the possible benefits of megadoses of vitamin C and the treatment of the common cold. The principal evidence for the protective benefits of high levels of vitamin C is anecdotal; the scientific evidence is virtually negative. One set of studies indicated, however, that 250 milligrams per day may be useful and cause no harm.

Cancer is another health problem in which vitamin C is thought to have some benefit. Though the claims are greatly exaggerated, a report issued by the National Academy of Science concluded that limited evidence suggests that vitamin C has been found to inhibit the formation of some carcinogens, and the consumption of vitamin C-containing foods is associated with a lower risk of stomach and esophageal cancer. The established allowances (RDAs) take into consideration the amount thought to be necessary for cancer prevention.

STRATEGIES

FOOD SOURCES Red peppers may be the richest source of vitamin C, certainly among vegetables. Other excellent choices are leafy green vegetables, brussels sprouts, broccoli, green peppers, potatoes, cabbage, and parsley. Turnips, cauliflower, collards, and spinach are also suitable. Citrus fruits are excellent sources, as are cantaloupe, papaya, strawberries, and tomatoes.

On the other hand, carrots, eggplant, lettuce, and celery are not good sources, nor are apples, grapes, pears, plums, and watermelon. Liver is the only animal food that is considered a significant source.

In the average American diet, fruits and vegetables supply 92 percent of all vitamin C, while meats, fish, poultry, eggs, and dairy products contribute about 8 percent.

Vitamin C is not evenly distributed among all the vegetables of a particular type or even in any one vegetable. The soil and conditions under which vegetables and fruits are grown, and how they are brought to market, will determine how much vitamin C they contain. Thin-stemmed vegetables fare better than thick-stemmed ones, and vegetables that wilt lose more vitamin C, and more quickly, than those that do not. The broccoli head has more vitamin C than the stem, but the stem retains more of its vitamin content than the head when cooked.

FOOD PREPARATION Because vitamin C is the most easily destroyed of all the vitamins, extra precautions must be taken to preserve the vitamin content of food while cooking. Losses occur when the food is exposed to air (oxidized), heat, and water (because they are water-soluble). Some foods protect their vitamin contents more effec-tively than others. Because of their large surface areas, for example, leafy vegetables lose more vitamin C in storage (oxidation) than root vegeta-bles. If the market stores vegetables in a refrigerated area or keeps them under crushed ice, this will reduce their vitamin loss.

Though it may be virtually impossible to know the condition in which the fruits and vegetables you purchase were grown and harvested, it is safe to assume that most are picked early (green) in order to reach you, the retail customer, when ripening. This is important because there is considerably more vitamin C in fruits and vegetables that are sun-ripened on the plant. When picked early or grown in the shade, they draw less vitamins from the host plant or tree.

Not all cooking methods are the same when it comes to vitamin destruction, but the less water and heat used, the more the vitamin is saved in the process. If you are canning raw vegetables or fruits, a brief steaming will actually help retention because steam destroys the enzymes that increase the rate of vitamin destruction.

The speed at which foods are frozen, as well as cooked, will be decisive in vitamin retention. Foods that are quick- or flash-frozen are likely to retain more vitamin C than foods frozen more slowly. On the other hand, losses are greatest when foods are dried (for example, sun-dried tomatoes) because, in addition to the time necessary to dry them, their exposure to sunlight (off the vine) increases vitamin C destruction.

It is wisest to buy fresh fruit in quantities that assure they will be eaten within a day or two. Vitamin C is easily oxidized, which means that prolonged exposure to air will destroy the vitamin content. The fruits should be chilled immediately after purchase and kept cold and uncut until eaten. Most of the vitamin content in fruit is found in or immediately under the skin, so peeling the fruit will cause considerable loss. If they are to be peeled, do so immediately before serving.

Fruit juices are also subject to vitamin loss, but acidic juices such as orange and grapefruit can be left covered in the refrigerator for at least a week without significant vitamin loss. It helps to fill the juice container to the top because it reduces the amount of air in the bottle.

Cook the vegetables in as little water as possible and cook them covered; less exposure to heat hastens cooking time and reduces vitamin loss through evaporation. Do not soak fresh vegetables; this will leach vitamin C from them. It is prudent to salvage the liquid in canned vegetables for other cooking purposes because much of the water-soluble vitamin probably has been leached into it.

Frozen foods should not be left to thaw for long periods before cooking. Place them in a small amount of boiling water and let them thaw and cook at the same time.

SPECIAL ADVICE Cooking in unlined copper pots, brass and nickel alloy (monel) pots, and especially iron pots can destroy some of the vitamin C. The use of steam tables for keeping foods warm for any period will also increase vitamin C loss.

DRUG INTERACTIONS Aspirin will cause the body to retain less of the dietary vitamin C. Therefore, constant and heavy use of aspirins may lead to a vitamin C deficiency. Barbiturates, taken to reduce anxiety, increase the need for vitamin C because they decrease its effectiveness.

Corticosteroids, drugs used to reduce inflammation, increase the need for vitamin C for two reasons: They accelerate various reactions in the body that require vitamin C, and they accelerate the excretion of the vitamin. Oral contraceptives also increase the rate at which vitamin C is used.

Alcohol is a vitamin C antagonist. Unfortunately, one of the drugs designed to treat alcoholism, Paraldehyde, increases the rate that vitamin C is metabolized, which increases the need for the vitamin.

Tetracycline increases the body's rate of excretion of vitamin C. If the drug is taken for two weeks, it is likely to increase the risk of a vitamin C deficiency.

When taking any of these drugs, it is advisable to get 100 milligrams of vitamin C per day.

It has been speculated that sulfur drugs increase the need for vitamin C, but the clinical evidence is not clear on this matter.

THIAMIN (VITAMIN B1)

DESCRIPTION

The most important function of Vitamin B1 (otherwise known as thiamin) is its role in normal metabolism. Its primary job is to break down and convert carbohydrates into glucose. The glucose, which is a sugar, is the sole source of energy required by the brain and nervous system. An enzyme found in red blood cells, the liver, kidneys, and other tissues requires the presence of this vitamin. Thiamin also plays a role in promoting appetite and a proper functioning digestive tract, while a deficiency of the vitamin seems to affect cardiac function.

FOOD SOURCES

Excellent Sources: sunflower seeds (dry and hulled), pecans, roast pork, peanuts, green peas, bran flakes (40 percent bran), and ham

Good Sources: raw oysters, asparagus, beef liver, orange juice, oatmeal, spinach, baked potatoes, and broccoli

HIGH-RISK GROUPS FOR POSSIBLE DEFICIENCY

- pregnant or breast-feeding women
- alcoholics
- people over 55
- people with wasting diseases
- people recovering from gastrointestinal surgery
- people with liver disease, chronic diarrhea, hyperthyroidism, and diabetes
- heavy users of aspirin
- heavy users of digitalis preparations (Crystodigin, Lanoxicaps, Lanoxin), a drug taken to increase the force with which the heart pumps
- heavy users of Mercurial Diuretics (Diamox, Daranide, Neptazane), a drug that reduces fluid retention and is commonly used in treatment of glaucoma

RECOMMENDED DOSAGE

GROUP	MG	GROUP	MG
Pregnant women	1.4	Children 7–10	1.2
Lactating women	1.5	Young women 11–22	1.1
Infants 0–.6	0.3	Adult women 23+	1.0
0.6–1	0.5	Young men 11–18	1.4
Children 1–3	0.7	19–22	1.5
4–6	0.9	Adult men 23–50	1.4
		51+	1.2

UPPER LIMITS FOR REGULAR DIETARY SUPPLEMENTAL USE

Children under 4 years of age: 1 mg
Adults and children 4 or more years of age: 3.0 mg
Pregnant or lactating women: 3 mg

BENEFITS

TREATING DEFICIENCY SYMPTOMS

MILD DEFICIENCY

- fatigue
- apathy
- loss of knee jerk
- numbness in the legs
- moodiness
- irritability
- gastrointestinal disorders
- loss of appetite
- constipation
- mild depression

GROSS DEFICIENCY

- heart enlargement
- tingling pain in the arms or legs
- edema in arms and legs
- atrophied muscles
- loss of weight
- paralysis in the lower extremities
- heart failure

OTHER POSSIBLE BENEFITS

- aids in treatment of herpes zoster
- aids in treatment of alcoholic cirrhosis
- aids in treatment of hyperactive thyroid
- aids in vitamin deficiency problems related to breast-feeding
- aids in vitamin deficiency problems associated with pregnancy

UNPROVEN BENEFITS (UNRELATED TO DEFICIENCY SYMPTOMS)

- cures depression
- acts as an analgesic
- protects against normal fatigue
- effective mosquito repellent (taken orally)
- aids in nervous disorders

TOXIC SYMPTOMS

Large doses may cause drowsiness (very rare).

DISCOVERY Though the existence of vitamin B1 was confirmed in the early 1900s, scientific proof of the existence of a group of

B vitamins waited until the 1920s. The identification of the separate B vitamins came only when scientists deduced the chemical structure of B1 (thiamin). Once this mystery was solved, biochemists were able to identify the structure of B2 (riboflavin), B3 (niacin), and the others. In terms of the fat-soluble vitamins, the Bs were late arrivals since the last two were discovered as late as 1945 (folacin) and 1948 (B12).

Much like the story of vitamin D and rickets (caused by a deficiency of vitamin D), the discovery of vitamin B1 is also tied to a disease, beriberi, a disease that produces symptoms of profound weakness due to a gross deficiency of vitamin B1.

Beriberi was a significant health problem among the sailors of the Indian navies during the eighteenth and nineteenth centuries. In that part of the world the life of sailors was harsh. Besides the rigors of life at sea, their diets were erratic, sometimes barely adequate. For weeks, possibly months, their diets might consist of little more than polished rice. Over time, such restricted diets caused the men to become profoundly weak, the classic symptoms of a vitamin B1 deficiency. In many cases it resulted in death.

As early as 1880 a Dutch naval doctor reported that death from beriberi was greatly reduced in Indian crews when European-type diets were provided instead of diets consisting primarily of polished rice. At about the same time a Japanese doctor wrote that beriberi had been eradicated among the sailors under his command when he added extra meat, fish, and vegetables to their regular diet. Before this time beriberi was so common that three out of every ten sailors were likely to have it, and it was a principal cause of death for merchant sailors in that part of the world.

Reaching the conclusion that beriberi was a diet-deficient disease was not an easy task. What stalled that conclusion was the presence of Louis Pasteur's germ theory. Germs were widely accepted as the principal, if not universal, explanation for the cause of most diseases. Consequently, it was understandable that medical researchers in the late nineteenth century thought microorganisms probably were the cause of beriberi. As a result, research scientists looked in vain for the responsible organism they were sure lurked somewhere beneath their microscopes.

The formal discovery of the cause of beriberi was by a Dutch physician named Christiaan Eijkman. In 1896 Dr. Eijkman observed that chickens being used in his laboratory for bacterial research showed symptoms similar to beriberi. He eventually learned that the chickens developed these symptoms only if they were fed polished rice from the kitchen; when fed unpolished or raw rice with the hull intact, they were cured of the beriberi.

He did not fully understand the significance of his specific discovery at the time. Initially, he thought the hull of the rice contained some substance that neutralized a naturally-occurring toxin in the rice. He believed the polished rice was virtually poisoning the chickens and the sailors.

Within the decade other biochemists determined that it was not what the polished rice contained but what it did not contain that caused the disease. They rightly deduced that the hull of the rice contained a missing food component necessary to a healthy life and that beriberi was another dietary deficiency disease. In other words, animals and humans could become diseased from a diet missing some essential component usually found naturally in only the smallest amounts and in only some foods.

For his general work in the new field of biochemical diseases and especially vitamin B1, Dr. Eijkman shared the Nobel Prize in 1929 with Sir Frederick Hopkins, the discoverer of vitamin D.

ROLE The most important function of vitamin B1 is sustaining the life of individual cells throughout the body. All of our body tissues depend on the energy that comes from the oxidation of the carbohydrates in our diet. Enzymes and their partners, nonprotein molecules called coenzymes, bring about the chemical changes that break down or oxidize the carbohydrates. Thiamin is critical to this whole process because it is part of the chemical structure of the enzyme thiamin pyrophosphate, which is an essential link in the energy production chain that oxidizes carbohydrates and feeds the body.

Many people mistakenly assume that since an increase of a vitamin corrects the symptoms of its deficiency, the vitamin will somehow correct the underlying causes that produce similar symptoms. They argue that since a thiamin deficiency can cause mild depression and thiamin supplements can eliminate that symptom, thiamin can treat other causes of depression as well.

PROBLEMS OF TOO LITTLE VITAMIN B1
One important property of thiamin is its water solubility. Unlike fat-soluble vitamins, which are stored in fat, the body is not capable of storing more than a one- or two-week supply of thiamin. The unused portion of our dietary thiamin is dissolved in the fluids of the body and excreted in the urine. The significance of this phenomenon is that we can become easily deficient if our diet does not consistently provide a proper amount of the vitamin. Conversely, megadoses are of little value because the body cannot store the vitamin to any extent. What the body is unable to use, which is only a limited amount, is excreted.

Our diet certainly provides enough thiamin to prevent any occurrence of beriberi, which occurs only with a gross thiamin deficiency. Unfortunately, beriberi is still prevalent in those parts of the world that rely on rice as its stable food.

Unfortunately, few foods in our diets are naturally rich in thiamin, which may account for the surveys that indicate the average diet in the United States provides little more than the recommended allowance. Studies indicate that the people whose diets are poor in thiamin (levels close to or less than the recommended allowance) and high in carbohydrates are at risk of deficiency symptoms such as loss of appetite, apathy, or fatigue.

The reason that more of us don't experience thiamin deficiency symptoms is due in large part to the enrichment of our foods with synthetic vitamins; breads and cereals fortified with vitamin B1 alone have increased our thiamin protection by about one-third.

WHO IS AT RISK   An inadequate diet can be the cause of a thiamin deficiency, especially for those who have an increased demand for the vitamin. People suffering from fevers or recovering from surgical operations frequently have a need for more thiamin. The elderly who reduce their diets to 2,000 or fewer calories may be placing themselves at such a risk. Studies also suggest that older persons may use thiamin less efficiently. Others who experience increased needs for thiamin are pregnant and lactating women; the lactating mother, in particular, needs as much as one and one-half times more thiamin.

To meet their high-energy demands, children routinely have greater thiamin needs in order to break down and convert their carbohydrates into glucose. Similar high-energy needs in young men explain why they require the same thiamin levels as lactating women.

Chronic alcoholics frequently experience nervous symptoms due to a lack of vitamin B1 because their diets are poor. Excessive alcohol, an antithiamin agent, reduces the absorption of thiamin and therefore increases the risk of a thiamin deficiency.

STRATEGIES

FOOD SOURCES   Although most natural foods contain thiamin, the amount supplied by any one given food is relatively small. Most fruits, for example, provide less than 5 percent of our dietary thiamin. Those foods that contain the most thiamin are whole grains, organ meats, lean pork, nuts, and legumes. Unlike milk fortified with vitamin D, no single food in our diet can be relied upon to supply a major portion of our thiamin needs. The obligation must be borne by our entire diet, which is an argument for a mixed diet.

Our total thiamin intake is distributed in approximately these percentages: about 41 percent comes from bread and cereals; 30 percent from meats, fish, poultry, and eggs; 7 percent from vegetables (especially tomatoes); 5 percent from dry beans, peas, and nuts; 5 percent from potatoes and sweet potatoes; 4 percent from fruits (especially citrus); and 8 percent from milk and other dairy products.

Sucrose (sugar) and pure fat that are used in processing certain foods and supply over 35 percent of the energy intake of an average American diet contain absolutely *no* thiamin (or other water-soluble vitamins, for that matter). Less inviting choices for your family's needs but a low-cost alternative to fast foods or highly processed foods are oatmeal, peas, and beans, which are rich in thiamin.

FOOD PREPARATION   Vitamin B1 is a water-soluble vitamin and is found in only minor amounts in most foods. It is reduced in food preparation, especially if the foods are boiled and the water discarded. If boiled, the amount of thiamin lost will vary depending on the length of cooking period and the amount of surface area exposed. If the pots are uncovered, evaporation will carry off some thiamin. This is a good argument for steaming thiamin-containing foods in covered pots so that far less of the vitamin will be lost.

Thiamin loss also occurs in high heat during home preparation, such as boiling ready-cooked cereal or toasting bread. At the same time, if you prepare cereals in a double boiler, especially if it is covered, there will be little vitamin loss. You shouldn't hesitate to blanch vegetables or stir-fry them, since cooking time is relatively brief. Again, it is prolonged exposure to heat that causes damage to the vitamin.

SPECIAL ADVICE   The choice of how you cook your meats will determine how much or how little thiamin is lost. Roasting meat may result in a 50 percent loss of thiamin, while broiling may lose only 30 percent and frying about 15 percent. When thawing frozen meats, save the drippings for gravy because they contain some of the thiamin lost in the process.

POOR FOOD SOURCES   Canned vegetables are a poor source of thiamin because the fluid in the can, which contains the thiamin that has been leached from the vegetables, is usually thrown away. Thiamin is also unstable in alkaline solutions; therefore, foods cooked with baking soda will lose significant amounts of the vitamin.

DRUG INTERACTIONS   Anyone taking Digitalis Preparations (Crystodigin, Lanoxicaps, Lanoxin), drugs taken to increase the force with which the heart pumps, may need an increase in vitamin B1. This same caution extends to anyone who uses Mercurial Diuretics (Diamox, Daranide, Neptazane), drugs commonly used in the treatment of glaucoma, because they can cause a vitamin B1 deficiency over time. Finally, constant use of aspirin can conceivably cause a deficiency because aspirin increases the excretion of thiamin.

RIBOFLAVIN (VITAMIN B2)

DESCRIPTION

The primary function of riboflavin (vitamin B2) is the metabolism of proteins, carbohydrates, and fats for energy production. It is also an essential component of living cells since riboflavin makes it possible for oxygen to reach the cells. In addition, riboflavin contributes to the growth and repair of the cell tissue throughout the body, especially of the skin, mucous membranes, and eyes.

FOOD SOURCES

Excellent sources: brewer's yeast, liver, heart, and kidney meats, milk, sardines, and cheese
Good sources: eggs, lean meats, leafy green vegetables, whole grain and enriched cereals

RISK GROUPS FOR POSSIBLE DEFICIENCY

- pregnant or breast-feeding women
- alcoholics and other drug abusers
- people over 55 years
- people with wasting diseases
- people whose daily diet is primarily processed foods
- people recovering from gastrointestinal surgery or severe burns
- women taking oral contraceptives
- people who participate in vigorous physical work
- people who take the drug Busulfan (Myleran) or Doxorubicin Hydrochloride (Adriamycin), drugs used in the treatment of cancer
- people who take Daunorubicin Hydrochloride (Cerubidine), an antileukemia drug
- people who take Chlorpromazine Hydrochloride (Thorazine)
- people who take Chloramphenicol (Chloromycetin) and Tetracycline, antibiotic drugs

RECOMMENDED DOSAGE

GROUP	MG	GROUP	MG
Pregnant women:	1.5	Infants 0.6–1	0.6
Lactating women:	1.7	Children 1–3	0.8
Infants 0–0.6	0.4	4–6	1.0

GROUP	MG	GROUP	MG
Children 7–10	1.4	Young men 15–22	1.7
Young women 11–22	1.3	Adult men 23–50	1.6
Adult women 23+	1.2	51+	1.4
Young men 11–14	1.6		

UPPER LIMITS FOR REGULAR DIETARY SUPPLEMENTAL USE
Children under 4 years of age: 1.2 mg
Adults and children 4 or more years of age: 2.6 mg
Pregnant or lactating women: 3.4 mg

TOXIC LEVELS
No toxic levels have been established.

BENEFITS
TREATING DEFICIENCY SYMPTOMS
- fissures at the angle of the mouth
- yellow crust in the corners of the mouth
- sensitivity to light
- painful red or purplish tongue
- trembling
- dizziness
- bloodshot or itching eyes
- damage to the cornea of the eye

OTHER POSSIBLE BENEFITS
- treatment of diseases of the liver
- treatment of infections
- treatment of stomach problems
- treatment of some clinic symptoms associated with alcoholism

UNPROVEN BENEFITS (UNRELATED TO DEFICIENCY SYMPTOMS)
- cures infertility
- improves poor vision
- promotes hair growth in men
- prevents cancer
- treats mononucleosis

TOXIC SYMPTOMS
Dark urine.

DISCOVERY   Before the turn of this century many people had suspected the existence of one soluble B vitamin, and between 1917 and 1927 researchers sensed there were at least two growth-promoting B vitamins in the foods they were studying—primarily liver, yeast, and the hulls of grains. The first real evidence of a second B vitamin occurred when yeast was heated long enough to destroy the thiamin (vitamin B1). What remained after the heat destroyed the thiamin was another substance that also showed growth-promoting properties. In 1927 the newest member of the family of B vitamins was scientifically confirmed and was named vitamin B2. (In the years that followed, biochemists subsequently learned the existence of more B vitamins.)

The story of the discovery of B vitamins becomes central to our entire understanding of vitamin function at this point.

German chemists in 1933 found that rats grew faster when given a yellow compound that was isolated from egg white. They called this vitamin compound *ovoflavin* (*flavus* means yellow). The significance of this discovery was that ovoflavin proved to be much the same as the yellow pigment or flavoenzyme discovered in 1931 that was associated with the consumption of oxygen in cell tissue. In other words, this was the first demonstration that linked vitamins with enzyme activity, clarifying the function of vitamins and opening the door to modern nutritional biochemistry.

In 1935 Dr. Paul Karrer (see Vitamin A, page 50) established that the yellow pigments isolated from foods as diverse as eggs, milk, and liver were all similar. In the same year he synthesized the vitamin (until then referred to only as vitamin B2) and gave it the name riboflavin.

ROLE   Riboflavin, found in both enzymes and coenzymes, plays an important role in a long and complicated chain of chemical reactions that support the life of cell tissues. Dr. Paul Karrer established that the principal function of riboflavin and its partner enzymes was to pass along the hydrogen atoms to a point where they are united with oxygen atoms to form water molecules. In this manner oxygen is delivered to the cell tissues and life is sustained.

PROBLEMS OF TOO LITTLE   Because riboflavin is essential for the conduct of many chemical reactions in skin tissues, if a deficiency occurs it will damage many different types of skin tissue; for example, a low dietary intake of riboflavin can cause *cheilosis* (in Greek *cheilos* means lip), which is dry skin around the nose and lips, and cracks or fissures at the angle of the mouth. A yellow crust will often form. It may also cause a condition called *glossitis* (in Greek *glossa* means tongue), which produces a painful and purplish red tongue. In some cases of a riboflavin deficiency the skin on the scrotum has become inflamed, and in others it has caused damage to the cornea of the eye, making it sensitive to light.

Riboflavin deficiency symptoms are relatively uncommon among most Americans, thanks to a program of food enrichment that was started by the Food and Drug Administration (FDA) in 1941. Before this time riboflavin deficiency was fairly common in the United States, especially in the South, and wherever milk, the most convenient dietary source of riboflavin, was not consumed in adequate quantities.

The principal reason for the uneven consumption of riboflavin in this country is that 15 to 25 percent of Americans use milk sparingly, if at all. Since milk (or dairy products) provides about 40 percent of the riboflavin consumed in the United States, it is apparent that people who do not consume milk must either rely on generous quantities of liver, eggs, leafy vegetables, and legumes, or take vitamin supplements to maintain an adequate intake.

WHO IS AT RISK   Minor deficiencies of riboflavin are most likely to occur in people with an inadequate intake of basic or enriched foods. Alcoholics are guilty of the kind of poor eating habits that lead to problems associated with riboflavin deficiencies, as are people over the age of sixty-five. People whose caloric intake is less than 2,000 calories are frequently deficient in vitamin B2.

Pregnant women are known to be at risk as well as young women of lower socioeconomic levels who are of childbearing age. Studies show that poor people generally eat inadequate diets, or at least diets that rely on fast foods, which are generally low in riboflavin.

Infants are generally well protected against a deficiency of riboflavin because both breast milk and cow's milk are excellent sources of riboflavin.

STRATEGIES

FOOD SOURCES   Unlike dairy products, which are the principal sources of our dietary calcium, no one food in our diet can meet most of our riboflavin needs. Both riboflavin and thiamin are widely distributed among many of the foods we commonly eat. The notable exceptions are pure sugars and fats, which contain no riboflavin or thiamin whatsoever.

Vitamins B2 and B1 are not distributed in foods in the same proportions. You will find more riboflavin in foods such as liver, kidneys, green leafy vegetables, and milk than vitamin B1. In fact, milk has about four times as much riboflavin as thiamin. On the other hand, whole cereals, which are just about the best source of thiamin we know, have only modest amounts of riboflavin. Beans, peas, nuts, and eggs are good sources of both vitamins, as are muscle meats (as opposed to organ meats). The one exception is pork meat, which has five to seven times the thiamin content of other foods but doesn't contain any more riboflavin than most other meats. This kind of distribution is another argument for the merits of a mixed diet containing meat, green vegetables, and dairy products.

As with so many nutrients (including thiamin, niacin, and iron), riboflavin has been added to our foods, especially breads and cereal products, as part of the government-sponsored enrichment program.

Our total riboflavin intake is distributed as follows: about 40 percent from milk and other dairy products (except butter); 27 percent from meats, fish, poultry, and eggs; 22 percent from bread and cereals; 5 percent from vegetables (especially tomatoes); 2 percent from nuts, dry beans, and peas; 2 percent from potatoes and sweet potatoes; and 2 percent from fruits (especially citrus).

Like most of the water-soluble vitamins, riboflavin is sensitive to light. If exposed to light during cooking—for example, if prepared in an open vessel—losses can occur. Vitamin loss also occurs if you use sodium bicarbonate in cooking vegetables. It is estimated that during their preparation as much as 20 percent of the riboflavin is lost in meats, maybe an average of 15 percent in vegetables, and 10 percent in baking bread.

Our understanding of how the vitamin can be destroyed through exposure to light has changed the way we package certain foods, especially the most important source of riboflavin in our diet. In 1960 we began to market milk in opaque cartons so that the milk would be protected from unnecessary exposure to light. It is believed that in home delivery a clear bottle of milk left standing for less than two hours on the doorstep in direct sunlight lost more than half of its riboflavin value. Even the display lighting in a dairy store caused vitamin loss when the milk was packaged in clear bottles.

DRUG INTERACTIONS   The drug Busulfan (Myleran) is an anticancer agent that prevents the formation of new cells, including healthy and unhealthy ones. It also prevents the absorption of nutrients through the lining of the intestine. For these two reasons, Busulfan can cause a riboflavin deficiency (as well as other vitamin deficiencies).

The antileukemia drug Daunorubicin Hydrochloride (Cerubidine) and another anticancer agent, Doxorubicin Hydrochloride (Adriamycin), are drugs that impair the conversion of riboflavin to its active form, resulting in a potential vitamin deficiency.

Antibiotic drugs such as Chloramphenicol (Chloromycetin) and the antipsychotic drug Chlorpromazine Hydrochloride (Thorazine) may cause a riboflavin deficiency because these drugs increase the need for more of the vitamin than is normal. Tetracycline, a commonly used antibiotic, can cause a deficiency over time because it increases the excretion of the vitamin.

It is believed that women who take oral contraceptives (containing estrogen) are at risk of a vitamin deficiency because estrogen stimulates reactions in the body that increase the need for riboflavin.

If you are taking these drugs, it is advised that you include milk in some form in every meal for the needed riboflavin. On the other hand, riboflavin supplements that greatly exceed RDA levels are not recommended because they can make the drugs less effective.

NIACIN (VITAMIN B3)

DESCRIPTION

Niacin (known also as nicotinamide, nicotinic acid, and vitamin B3) is a vitamin that is essential to providing energy for cell tissue growth. Working with two separate enzymes, niacin provides the energy to cell tissue by oxidizing glucose. Along with thiamin and riboflavin, this vitamin plays an important role in the metabolism of carbohydrates and contributes to the maintenance of healthy tissue growth of the skin, mucous membranes, and the digestive system.

FOOD SOURCES

Excellent sources: roasted peanuts, chicken, beef liver, turkey, tuna, salmon, sunflower seeds, and raw oysters

Good sources: peas, beans, apricots, whole-grain or enriched cereals, potatoes, and collards

HIGH RISK GROUPS FOR POSSIBLE DEFICIENCY

- pregnant or breast-feeding women
- alcoholics and other drug abusers
- people over 55
- people with wasting diseases
- people suffering from hyperthyroidism
- people recovering from gastrointestinal surgery or severe burns
- people who participate in vigorous physical work
- people who take the drug Busulfan (Myleran) that is used in the treatment of cancer
- people who take Isoniazid (INH, Rifamate), a drug for treating tuberculosis
- people who take Mercaptopurine (Purinethol), an antileukemia drug
- people who take Levodopa (Larodopa, Sinemet), a drug for treating Parkinson's disease

RECOMMENDED DOSAGE

GROUP	MG	GROUP	MG
Pregnant women	15	Children 7–10	16
Lactating women	16	Young women 11–14	15
Infants 0–0.6	6	15–22	14
0.6–1	8	Adult women 23+	13
Children 1–3	9	Young men 11–18	18
4–6	11	19–22	19
		Adult men 23–50	18
		51+	16

UPPER LIMITS FOR REGULAR DIETARY SUPPLEMENTAL USE

Children under 4 years of age: 13.5 mg
Adults and children 4 or more years of age: 30 mg
Pregnant or lactating women: 40 mg

TOXIC LEVELS

Unknown.

BENEFITS

TREATING DEFICIENCY SYMPTOMS OF
- general fatigue
- loss of appetite
- skin disorders (especially on parts exposed to sun)
- diarrhea
- irritability
- mouth swelling
- smooth tongue
- mental confusion

OTHER POSSIBLE BENEFITS
- treatment of premenstrual cramps
- dilates blood vessels
- reduces blood cholesterol (with the use of 1,000 to 2,000 milligrams under strict medical supervision)
- treatment of vertigo

UNPROVEN BENEFITS (UNRELATED TO DEFICIENCY SYMPTOMS)

- cures depression
- improves poor digestion
- stimulates sex drive
- reduces high blood pressure

TOXIC SYMPTOMS

Flushing of the skin, vomiting, abdominal cramps, diarrhea, headache, and sweating.

DISCOVERY   The discovery of many of the individual vitamins came as a result of research on a number of diseases. In most cases it was learned that the cause of the disease was something missing from the daily diet of the patient. Two examples would be the disease of rickets (caused by a deficiency in vitamin D) and beriberi (caused by a deficiency in vitamin B1). By the end of the nineteenth century, biochemical researchers were referring to a new class of diseases called "diet deficient diseases." In this regard the story of niacin, or what had been called vitamin B3, is much the same.

Pellagra is a disease that was commonly seen among the poor in the seventeenth and eighteenth centuries. Its most identifying symptom is a reddish skin rash that causes the skin to dry, crack, and peel. When exposed to the sun, the skin becomes dark and rough. The progress of the disease has been termed the four Ds: dermatitis, diarrhea, dementia, and death.

At the turn of this century Louis Pasteur's germ theory dominated the thinking about the causes of human disease. It was almost universally accepted that microorganisms, called germs, caused most diseases, and for good measure, they explained how diseases were communicated (communicable diseases). Many observers came to believe that pellagra was caused by germs or some toxic substance found in the diet of the people affected.

In 1907 an epidemic of pellagra broke out in the southern part of the United States, and by 1917 more than two hundred thousand cases were reported throughout the country. In Lombardy the doctors believed that spoiled corn, which the peasants used to make polenta or cornmeal porridge, caused the epidemic. In the southern United States, where the poor sharecroppers and mill hands live almost exclusively on cornmeal and grits, opinion as to the cause of the pellagra was divided between toxic corn and an infection. The corn eater theory was understandable because the disease had appeared most often among people whose diet consisted mostly of corn.

Working for the U. S. Public Health Service, a biochemist, Dr. Joseph Goldberger, studied the problem and concluded that instead of being an infectious disease or one caused by toxic corn, pellagra was caused by a missing food factor. Others had suspected that pellagra was caused by a poor diet, but Goldberger was the first to identify certain foods that contained substances which seemingly prevented the disease. Goldberger called this the P-P factor (pellagra-preventive) and believed it to be the new vitamin find at the time, vitamin B2 or riboflavin. It proved later to be a new vitamin, niacin or vitamin B3.

The work of another American biochemist, Dr. Conrad Elvehjem, determined that nicotinic acid, or nicotinamide, was in fact Goldberger's missing food factor. In 1937 at the University of Wisconsin, Dr. Elvehjem showed that blacktongue—which is pellagra in dogs—could be cured by giving them nicotinic acid, a substance he had isolated from beef liver. (Vitamin B3 appears in two natural forms: nicotinic acid and nicotinamide. Niacin is a collective term for these two natural compounds. Compound vitamins, such as niacin, are often referred to as *vitaminers,* which is the term that characterizes any of two or more compounds that relieve a deficiency of a specific vitamin.)

The latest chapter of the niacin story is fairly recent since it was not until 1945 that biochemists discovered the body used an amino acid, tryptophan, to produce nicotinic acid. In fact, they learned that in sufficient amounts dietary tryptophan could overcome the symptoms of pellagra without the assistance of dietary niacin.

ROLE   What we know about the many functions of vitamins is drawn from what we see when there is a gross deficiency of the vitamin. In the case of niacin we know that a deficiency initially damages skin tissue and then the cell tissue of the gastrointestinal tract and nervous system. The symptoms, if unchecked, follow the same course: first a skin rash, then persistent diarrhea, and finally dementia and possibly death.

Niacin is found in all tissues of the body but especially in the liver, kidney, heart, brain, and muscles. As with vitamins B1 and B2, the principal function of niacin is in the oxidative process of the living cell. Without these three vitamins, B1, B2, and B3, the coenzymes designed to transport hydrogen could not function. Thiamin, riboflavin, and niacin all work with enzymes and coenzymes to form a long and complicated chain of chemical reactions that release energy from glucose (once it is metabolized from our foods) and with their partner enzymes pass along hydrogen atoms to a point where they are united with oxygen atoms to form water molecules.

PROBLEMS OF TOO LITTLE   There is little evidence showing how a niacin deficiency provokes the symptoms that it does. Part of the answer may lie in the fact that pellagra seldom exists without deficiencies in thiamin and riboflavin. Usually, when niacin is administered along with other B vitamins, the symptoms of the deficiency disappear. Of course, the symptoms anyone might experience will depend on the gravity of their niacin deficiency.

Symptoms of a very mild niacin deficiency may be difficult to identify at first. One early sign is a sore tongue. It may later become red and perhaps swollen, and then the mouth may grow progressively sorer. If the deficiency continues, it is common for the gastrointestinal tract to get inflamed and for diarrhea to occur.

The principal and most dramatic symptom of pellagra is dermatitis. The skin becomes reddish, especially on the face, hands, and feet, and when the rash is exposed to the sunlight, it becomes dark and rough. Peculiar to pellagra, the rash appears almost always on both sides of the body at the same time. In addition to a very sore mouth and tongue, the aggravated lining of the digestive tract may produce bloody diarrhea that results in a loss of weight, anemia, and dehydration. In a later stage, though it is more likely someone with the deficiency would receive medical attention before reaching this stage, there will be a change in behavior such as anxiety and depression; in advanced cases there is confusion and stupor.

Our source for niacin is not restricted to food rich in the vitamin. As we said earlier, biochemists in 1945 learned that niacin can be made in the tissues of the body from the amino acid tryptophan. It was not necessary, therefore, to stress foods rich in niacin or niacin supplements as the only protection against pellagra. Since the body can form niacin from the amino acid tryptophan, which in turn can duplicate the same function as niacin, some foods rich in tryptophan but poor sources of niacin, such as milk and eggs, are also capable of preventing pellagra.

What biochemists learned from this discovery was that pellagra occurs only if the diet is poor in both niacin and tryptophan. Corn was implicated early on because corn was a poor source of both niacin and tryptophan and it was a diet staple. The following table gives you some idea of how a diet made up primarily of a staple such as wheat would not have caused pellagra, whereas corn could—and did.

Food	Quantity	Tryptophan	Niacin
Whole corn	100 gm	55 mg	2.0 mg
Whole wheat	100 gm	168 mg	4.3 mg

SYNTHESIS Determining how much niacin should be in our diets is further complicated by the fact that biochemists have learned that, like vitamins K and B1, niacin is also synthesized by bacteria in the intestine of the body. This bacterial synthesis does not produce great quantities of the vitamin, but it can be decisive in preventing pellagra or niacin deficiency symptoms if the diet is providing only borderline quantities of niacin and tryptophan. A diet that stresses vegetables is more suitable for this synthesis than most meat diets.

WHO IS AT RISK In the years before World War II pellagra was still a community health issue in certain parts of the country, but once we came to understand the health problems associated with a one-crop diet and mounted major public health education programs toward eating a mixed diet, pellagra became virtually nonexistent in the United States. In some parts of the world, however, where a highly milled flour or rice is consumed as the principal staple, pellagra still flourishes.

Though they are relatively uncommon, some few cases continue to be reported in the United States. Pellagra appears among some chronic alcoholics who have substituted alcohol for food over many months. People who have gone on severe low-calorie diets that restrict intake of protein, vitamins, and minerals will occasionally show symptoms. Pellagra is also one of those diet-deficient diseases that can be caused by another underlying disease or disorder that interferes with the normal absorption or utilization of food; for example, pellagra can be caused by chronic diarrhea, cirrhosis, hyperthyroidism, and tuberculosis.

Though we have seen the demise of pellagra as a disease in this country, we still have the problem of low-grade niacin deficiencies. People with poor niacin levels may not routinely show any symptoms, but if their need for niacin increases, their meager vitamin stores may be inadequate to meet the increased demand. For example, people taking certain medications that either interfere with the absorption or the utilization of niacin and people with wasting diseases or recovering from intestinal surgery (which may cause temporary food absorption problems) may begin to show signs of a niacin deficiency. Pregnant women and nursing mothers may also find a temporary need for more niacin in their diet. Some athletes and those who work out strenuously have learned that their niacin-poor diets poorly prepare them for their demanding work.

STRATEGIES

FOOD SOURCES   Since niacin can be formed in the body with the help of tryptophan, a diet requiring good food sources of niacin should include foods rich in tryptophan. In some cases they are the same foods. Heading the list of excellent niacin and tryptophan foods is roasted peanuts (peanut butter). Sunflower seeds are also very good. Other foods naturally rich in both tryptophan and niacin are liver, lean meat, fish, and poultry.

To prevent a niacin deficiency, legumes should be included in the diet because they are rich in all B vitamins. The list includes whole-grain cereals as well. It should be noted that breads and cereal products are good sources of niacin because the vitamin has been added to these foods as part of the government-sponsored enrichment program. Milk is on this recommended list of foods because it is a rich source of the necessary amino acid tryptophan.

Some foods are a surprise as to their restricted food values; for example, corn and rice, so important to diets all over the world, are extremely poor sources of niacin and tryptophan. And foods such as wheat germ and soybean and corn oils, which are some of the best-known sources of vitamin E in the world, are completely devoid of niacin.

Our total niacin intake is distributed in approximately these percentages: 45 percent from meats, fish, and poultry; about 28 percent from flour and cereal products; 8 percent from dry beans, peas, and nuts; 7 percent from potatoes and sweet potatoes; 5 percent from tomatoes and vegetables (excluding dark green and yellow vegetables); 2 percent from fruits (especially citrus); 2 percent from milk and other dairy products (except butter); and other foods 3 percent.

FOOD PREPARATION   Since niacin is not easily destroyed by exposure to air, light, and heat, most of the vitamin remains intact during normal cooking procedures. Like the other water-soluble vitamins, however, niacin can be lost in the drippings and juices of the meat. One good reason to make use of these drippings, in gravy for example, is that they could contain as much as 40 percent of the niacin after cooking.

DRUG INTERACTIONS   Busulfan (Myleran) is an anticancer agent that prevents the formation of new cells, healthy and unhealthy ones. It also prevents the absorption of nutrients through the lining of the intestine. For these two reasons, Busulfan can cause a niacin deficiency as well as other vitamin deficiencies.

The antitubercular drug Isoniazid (INH and Rifamate) can cause vitamin B6 to excrete more quickly, making it less effective. Since vitamin B6 and niacin work interdependently, the B6 deficiency could lead to a niacin deficiency. These two vitamins are also affected by Levodopa (Larodopa and Sinemet), a drug used in the treatment of Parkinson's disease. The drug can create a B6 deficiency by binding to the drug and making both the drug and the vitamin less effective. This binding action can effect, ultimately, a niacin deficiency as well.

Mercaptopurine (Purinethol) is used in treating leukemia. It is not likely that it will cause a niacin deficiency, but cases have been reported. If your diet is poor in niacin, therefore, you may be at some risk of a deficiency.

PYRIDOXINE (VITAMIN B6)

DESCRIPTION

Vitamin B6 is central to the work of probably more than fifty tasks in the body. It is involved in the absorption and metabolism of amino acids, the production of energy through the production of glucose, the formation of red blood cells, and the maintenance of the nervous system. It also plays a role in the formation of niacin (Vitamin B3) from tryptophan.

FOOD SOURCES

Excellent Sources: brewer's yeast, toasted wheat germ, sunflower seeds, beef liver, and soybeans
Good sources: bananas, avocados, chicken, fish, lean meats (for example, cooked veal), whole-grain cereals, nuts, spinach, potatoes, and leafy green vegetables

HIGH-RISK GROUPS FOR POSSIBLE DEFICIENCY

- pregnant and breast-feeding women
- heavy users of alcohol
- people recovering from gastrointestinal surgery or severe burns
- people suffering from a wasting disease
- anyone on a severe low-calorie diet
- women taking oral contraceptives or estrogen
- people over the age of 60
- people who take Busulfan (Myleran)
- people who take Chloramphenicol (Chloromycetin)
- people who take Levodopa (Larodopa and Sinemet)
- people who take Penicillamine (Cuprimine and Depen)
- people who take an antihypertensive drug called Hydralazine
- people who take antibiotics such as Tetracycline, Erythromycin, Lincomycin, and Neomycin
- people who take the antitubercular drugs Cycloserine (Seromycin), Para-Aminosalicylic Acid, Isoniazid (INH and Rifamate)
- people who take the antileukemia drug Chlorambucil (Leukeran)
- people who take Phenobarbital

RECOMMENDED DOSAGE

GROUP	MG	GROUP	MG
Pregnant women	2.6	Young Women 15–18	2.0
Lactating women	2.5	19–22	2.0
Infants 0–.6	0.3	Adult Women 23–50	2.0
.6–1	0.6	51 +	2.0
Children 1–3	0.9	Young Men 11–14	1.8
4–6	1.3	15–18	2.0
7–10	1.6	19–22	2.2
Young Women 11–14	1.8	Adult Men 23–50	2.2
		51+	2.2

UPPER LIMITS FOR REGULAR DIETARY SUPPLEMENTAL USE

Children under 4 years of age: 1 mg
Adults and children 4 or more years of age: 3 mg
Pregnant or lactating women: 4 mg

BENEFITS
TREATING DEFICIENCY SYMPTOMS

- anemia
- irritability
- nervousness
- insomnia
- breaks in the skin, especially around the eyes
- discolored or painful tongue
- difficulty walking
- kidney stones

OTHER POSSIBLE BENEFITS

- treatment of carpal tunnel syndrome (a disease that causes a paralysis of the fingers)
- treatment of nausea during pregnancy
- treatment of PMS symptoms

UNPROVEN BENEFITS (UNRELATED TO DEFICIENCY SYMPTOMS)

- aids in atherosclerosis
- aids in diabetes
- aids in arthritis
- relieves morning sickness
- aids in eye problems
- cures migraines
- prevents tooth decay
- acts as a tranquilizer

TOXIC SYMPTOMS

Numbness in the hands and feet.

DISCOVERY   In 1938, the year vitamin B6 was first isolated, the news was announced almost simultaneously in several different laboratories both in America and Europe. At the University of California, Berkeley, the vitamin was isolated and the three forms in which it naturally appears were given their names: pyridoxine, pyridoxal, and pyridoxamine. There is little difference among these three compounds that comprise vitamin B6. Once ingested and converted to the coenzyme pyridoxal phosphate, they all perform essentially the same metabolic functions.

Pyridoxal and pyridoxamine are the forms of vitamin B6 found in animals, and they are more easily absorbed; pyridoxine is present in plant foods and is more resistant to destruction by heat.

ROLE   Vitamin B6 performs many tasks in metabolism, especially those related to the breakdown of protein and amino acids.

Vitamin B6 creates from the amino acid three different hormones or hormonelike substances that are necessary to specific regulatory functions in the body. It is also essential for producing energy from the amino acids, and, along with other B vitamins, it is involved in the breakdown of glycogen to glucose for the production of energy. In fact, there are perhaps as many as fifty different activities that require the presence of vitamin B6 or its coenzyme pyridoxal phosphate.

In addition to the tasks already mentioned, vitamin B6 is a catalyst in the formation of niacin (vitamin B3) from tryptophan. Studies show that animals deficient in vitamin B6 cannot produce niacin, a fact that some researchers feel explains why symptoms of vitamin B6 deficiency are similar to those found in pellagra (see Vitamin B3, page 101).

Another relation exists between riboflavin (vitamin B2) and vitamin B6 since vitamin B2 appears to be involved in the conversion of pyridoxine into its active form. Such an arrangement suggests that a deficiency of riboflavin in the diet may lead to a deficiency of vitamin B6.

Vitamin B6 is also seen as important in protecting us from specific infections, especially genitourinary infections.

TOO LITTLE VITAMIN B6   Some of the deficiency symptoms of vitamin B6 are similar to those of vitamins B2 and B3, especially the dermatitis around the eyes and the painful and red tongue. If the deficiency is protracted, the symptoms may become severe and include dizziness, nausea, vomiting, loss of appetite, general weakness, irritability, and confusion. The deficiency can also produce kidney stones because during a vitamin B6 deficiency the amount of urinary citrate, a substance that aids in dissolving oxalate salts, is significantly reduced.

With the exception of the kidney stones, which would have to be treated separately, all of these symptoms will disappear once vitamin B6 is taken in sufficient quantities to correct the deficiency, perhaps as much as 5 milligrams daily.

One of the principal tasks of vitamin B6 is its role as a cofactor in the breakdown of protein. The more protein we eat, therefore, the more vitamin B6 we require. People who eat abnormally high amounts of protein may develop some symptoms of a vitamin B6 deficiency if their intake of B6 is marginal.

WHO IS AT RISK   The use of oral contraceptives apparently leads to changes similar to those of a B6 deficiency. Specifically, some clinicians point to depression during pregnancy that they attribute to a failure to convert tryptophan, which affects levels of serotonin, a substance produced in the brain that affects a wide range of behaviors, including sleep and moods.

Pregnancy may create a need for more vitamin B6. The fetus usually requires much higher levels of B6 than does the mother; the B6 levels of women who have suffered a toxemia of pregnancy were about one-third the normal amount. Vitamin B6 has also been used, with some success, for treating the nausea of pregnant women, but no theory has been accepted to explain why it works. In addition to pregnancy, people with long-term fevers may develop a deficiency because of the increase in metabolic activity brought on by the fever.

Some infants have become excessively irritable and convulsive when they have not received more than .1 milligram of vitamin B6 per day, but their symptoms almost always disappear as soon as the vitamin is added to their diet.

Those people who take a variety of prescription drugs may be at risk (see Drug Interactions, page 110), especially Isoniazid (used in the treatment of tuberculosis) and Penicillamine (used in treating Wilson's disease and rheumatoid arthritis).

NOTE   Breast milk is often deficient in B6 because it is believed that only about 4 percent of a mother's intake of vitamin B6 is made available to the baby through her own milk. Women who have used oral contraceptives for more than thirty months also have difficulty producing milk with sufficient B6 levels. In these circumstances they usually receive a supplement of 2.5 to 5 milligrams per day to correct the problem because it is rather difficult to reach 5 milligrams of vitamin B6 through dietary means alone. (Estimates as to the amount of vitamin B6 that is likely to appear in our normal diet vary from 1.7 to 2.3 milligrams daily per person.)

Certainly anyone who is unable to absorb vitamins properly is at risk. People who are recovering from gastrointestinal surgery may have some temporary difficulty absorbing vitamins and other nutrients, and those who have suffered from severe burns have an abnormal need for vitamin B6 as well.

It goes without saying that a poor diet is always a mild risk factor. Alcoholics, some who clinically starve themselves for brief periods, will frequently exhibit a vitamin B6 deficiency. This concern over the consequences of a poor diet applies also to those on a severe low-calorie diet and the elderly who often fail to eat properly.

STRATEGIES

FOOD SOURCES   In much the same manner as the other B vitamins, B6 is widely distributed throughout the foods we eat. To satisfy our nutrient needs for vitamin B6, our diet should contain foods such as whole-grain cereals, fish (especially salmon), chicken, liver, and egg yolks. Processed or refined foods such as white bread, spaghetti, macaroni, noodles and precooked rice are quite low in vitamin B6. Pure fat and sugar contain absolutely no vitamin B6, or other vitamins for that matter.

FOOD PREPARATION   B6 is relatively stable in heat but can be destroyed in sunlight (ultraviolet light). Freezing can cause upwards of a 70 percent vitamin loss, and the milling of wheat and other grains can lead to more than a 50 percent loss. Vitamin B6 is not a part of the white flour enrichment program and is generally not added to breads, as are some other B vitamins, but many cereals are fortified with the vitamin.

Food preparation in the home can contribute to the loss of vitamin B6 from our diet. Boiling foods in large quantities of water will increase the loss of this vitamin, and foods standing in a restaurant kitchen or cooked in water containing alkaloids will lose between 15 and 30 percent of their vitamin B6 contents.

TOO MUCH VITAMIN B6   Vitamin B6 is not very toxic, and some would say that for all practical purposes it is nontoxic. Because it is water soluble, if taken in large quantities the amount that is not used is excreted through the urine. Nevertheless, there have been some cases reported of B6 toxicity among individuals who had taken 200 to 600 milligrams over a two-month period.

Women taking oral contraceptives or pills containing estrogen have found that their deficiency symptoms disappear with daily supplements of 10 milligrams of vitamin B6. What should not be encouraged is the use of massive doses of B6 to treat symptoms resistant to modest amounts of vitamin B6. Reason would argue that these symptoms are probably unrelated to a B6 deficiency and should be treated by a physician. There is no reason either to take massive doses to "ward off" any future symptoms because vitamin B6 is water soluble and cannot be stored in the body. Symptoms that persist should be brought to the attention of your doctor.

DRUG INTERACTIONS   Busulfan (Myleran) is an agent that prevents the formation of healthy and unhealthy cells. It also prevents the absorption of nutrients through the lining of the intestine. For these two reasons, Busulfan can cause a vitamin B6 deficiency.

People who take corticosteroids, which are drugs that accelerate the reactions in the body, will need more than the normal amount of vitamin B6.

Cycloserine (Seromycin), Para-Aminosalicylic Acid, and Isoniazid (INH and Rifamate) cause vitamin B6 to be excreted more quickly, making it less effective. While taking these drugs, it might be advisable to take 5 milligrams of vitamin B6.

Chloramphenicol, Erythromycin, Lincomycin, and Neomycin are all antibiotic drugs that inactivate vitamin B6, making a vitamin B6 deficiency possible over time. Tetracycline inactivates vitamin B6 and could conceivably produce a deficiency in someone who is already at risk, such as heavy drinkers and women on oral contraceptives.

Oral contraceptives that contain estrogen and progestins stimulate many reactions in the body that require vitamin B6, including the breakdown of dietary protein. It is possible that the reduced production of serotonin due to vitamin B6 deficiency is responsible for depression while taking these drugs.

Hydralazine, an antihypertensive drug, significantly increases the excretion of vitamin B6, making a deficiency a distinct possibility. Phenobarbital, which is a sedative, impairs the absorption of a number of vitamins, including vitamin B6.

Vitamin B6 is also adversely affected by Levodopa (Larodopa and Sinemet), drugs used in the treatment of Parkinson's disease. The drug creates a B6 deficiency by binding to the vitamin and making both the drug and the vitamin less effective. Another drug that binds to vitamin B6 to prevent it from carrying out its normal functions is Penicillamine (Cuprimine and Depen). This drug, which is called a chelating agent, is used in the treatment of copper and lead poisoning because it binds to heavy metals and flushes them safely out of the body in the urine. Unfortunately, it also captures vitamin B6 and carries it out as well.

Penicillin inactivates vitamin B6, but a deficiency would occur only after long-term use. At risk are those who tend to have marginal deficiencies of the vitamin.

If you are using one of these drugs, a suitable preventive measure would be to take a 4-milligram supplement. If you are concerned about a deficiency because, in addition to using one of the above-mentioned drugs, you eat a poor diet or are recovering from gastrointestinal surgery or have some disorder that interferes with the absorption of vitamins, it may be prudent for you to take 5 milligrams daily during the risk period. There is no reason to take megadoses of vitamin B6, however, without the supervision of a doctor.

COBALAMIN (VITAMIN B12)

DESCRIPTION

Vitamin B12 is a water-soluble vitamin that is different from the other B vitamins in that it contains cobalt and other essential mineral elements. It is necessary to the functioning of all body cells, especially those of the bone marrow, nervous system, and gastrointestinal tract. Its main role is to aid in the formation of red blood cells and amino acids, and in the functioning of the nervous system. Fat, protein, and carbohydrate metabolism also depend on this vitamin, and it aids in the production of genetic materials—DNA and RNA.

FOOD SOURCES

Excellent sources: liver (especially lamb and beef), kidneys, raw clams, raw oysters, liverwurst, and herring
Good sources: canned sardines, canned crab, dehydrated cod, cheddar and cottage cheeses

HIGH-RISK GROUPS FOR POSSIBLE DEFICIENCY

- strict vegetarians
- heavy users of alcohol
- people recovering from gastrointestinal surgery or severe burns
- people suffering from a wasting disease
- anyone on a severe low-calorie diet
- women taking oral contraceptives
- people suffering from hypothyroidism
- people who take Methotrexate (Folex and Mexate)
- people who take Cholestyramine and Clofibrate (Atromid-S)
- people who take Penicillin
- people who take antibiotics such as Chloramphenicol (Chloromycin), Erythromycin, Sulfisoxazole, and Sulfamethoxazole
- people who take the antitubercular drugs Cycloserine (Seromycin), Para-Aminosalicylic Acid, Isoniazid (INH and Rifamate)
- people who take the antigout drug Colchicine

RECOMMENDED DOSAGE

GROUP	MCG	GROUP	MCG
Pregnant women	4.0	Children 7–10	3.0
Lactating women	4.0	Young women 11–14	3.0
Infants 0–.6	0.5	15–18	3.0
.6–1	1.5	Young women 19–22	3.0
Children 1–3	2.0	Adult women 23–50	3.0
4–6	2.5	51+	3.0
		Young men 11–14	3.0
		15–18	3.0
		19–22	3.0
		Adult men 23–50	3.0
		51+	3.0

UPPER LIMITS FOR REGULAR DIETARY SUPPLEMENTAL USE

Children under 4 years of age: 4.5 mcg
Adults and children 4 or more years of age: 9 mcg
Pregnant or lactating women: 12 mcg

BENEFITS

TREATING DEFICIENCY SYMPTOMS
(PERNICIOUS ANEMIA)
- bleeding gums
- gross fatigue
- sore tongue
- numbness and tingling in hands and feet
- pale lips, tongue, and gums
- depression
- shortness of breath
- nausea and loss of appetite

UNPROVEN BENEFITS (UNRELATED TO DEFICIENCY SYMPTOMS):

- treats allergies
- treats sterility
- treats thyroid disorders
- treats menstrual disorders
- treats eye problems
- treats headaches
- treats night blindness
- treats psoriasis and warts

TOXIC SYMPTOMS

Nosebleeds and dry mouth.

DISCOVERY   The last vitamin to be discovered was vitamin B12 in 1948. Once again, it was through the treatment of a diet deficiency disease that the discovery of this vitamin was made.

In the middle of the nineteenth century, an English physician named Thomas Addison provided a detailed description of the symptoms of a then incurable and fatal disease which we now know as pernicious ane mia. Aptly named, it resisted diagnosis and treatment for almost another one hundred years.

American physician George Richards Minot was interested in a blood disorder in which the red blood corpuscles steadily continued to die, usually with fatal consequences (pernicious anemia). Minot knew that early experiments established that eating beef liver could favorably affect the red blood corpuscle count. He concluded that pernicious anemia was a diet-deficient disease that must result from a lack of an unknown vitamin—a vitamin that must be present in significant quantities in liver.

In 1926 Dr. Minot his assistant, William Perry Murphy, another American physician, announced that eating as much as two-thirds of a pound of raw liver each day would favorably affect the level of red blood cells. One of the first benefits of their work was the development of liver products that could be fed to patients, eliminating the need for eating large amounts of raw liver—a disagreeable dietary task under most circumstances.

It was not an easy matter to identify this essential component that the liver contained since humans were the only creatures that displayed a need for the substance. Since pernicious anemia is not a disorder known to other animals, the usefulness of animal studies was limited. Consequently, over the years experiments were conducted on people already suffering from pernicious anemia to identify the elusive factor. In 1946 biochemists thought they had discovered the correct substance, but it was soon determined that folacin was not the antipernicious anemia factor they sought. Some of folacin's functions deal with the formation of nucleic acids (essential genetic growth factors in all animal life), and this role is very similar to the one played by vitamin B12.

Only two years later, in 1948, researchers in Britain and the United States simultaneously isolated this last vitamin—vitamin B12, now known also as cobalamin. (Vitamin B12 contains the mineral cobalt.)

To give you an idea of the newness of this vitamin, it was only in 1973 that vitamin B12 was synthesized. Its synthesis is expensive but, fortunately, vitamin manufacturers have been able to produce a vitamin B12 concentrate from cultures of certain bacteria and fungi grown in large tanks. It is these concentrates that constitute the vitamin B12 supplements so many people use.

ROLE   Once in the body vitamin B12 is converted to a coenzyme and is circulated in the blood, bound to one of several proteins. It is stored in the liver and kidneys of animals and humans, making organ meats of animals rich sources of vitamin B12. It is also found in the heart, pancreas, testes, brain, and bone marrow, areas of the body that are related to red blood formation.

The vitamin is central to the normal functioning of all cell tissue, especially of the bone marrow, nervous system, and gastrointestinal tract. Another very important role is in the formation of nucleic acids, leading to DNA and RNA formation. With the help of two other vitamins, choline and folacin, and a specific type of amino acid called methionine, vitamin B12 indirectly aids in the synthesis and metabolism of nerve and spinal cord tissue.

TOO LITTLE VITAMIN B12   The bad news is that only 30 to 70 percent of vitamin B12 is readily absorbed in even the most healthy person—and in the case of pernicious anemia, very little or none of it is absorbed. On the other hand, it appears that the need for vitamin B12 or cobalamin in humans is rather small and, when the intake is low, the body seems to conserve its stores of the vitamin by excreting less in the bile.

Successful absorption depends upon the presence of a protein enzyme referred to as a mucoprotein (muco is a form of the Latin mucus) that is secreted by specific cells in the wall of the stomach as a normal part of gastric juice. The mucoprotein normally binds to vitamin B12 and assists in its absorption from the gastrointestinal tract. But when autoimmune reactions make the enzyme unavailable along with other gastric secretions, the vitamin is not absorbed. This intrinsic factor that researchers discovered explained why pernicious anemia occurred among some people even though their diet seemed to supply adequate amounts of vitamin B12.

Absorption is also dependent upon the presence of calcium and hydrochloric acid in the gastrointestinal tract. Usually, anyone deficient in vitamin B12 either lacks one or more gastric secretions necessary for proper absorption or has an impaired thyroid gland.

Absorption also appears to be affected by the amount of vitamin B12 available. In other words, if your intake is low, absorption grows more efficient, reaching as high as 80 percent. But if higher amounts of it are consumed, the percentage absorbed drops to as little as perhaps 10 percent. What is significant about this phenomenon is that vitamin B12 absorption is improved when supplements are taken several times during the day instead of only once.

WHO IS AT RISK   Though deficiencies are somewhat rare, it may be a consideration for those who are strict vegetarians or "vegans," people who prefer to eat no animal products whatsoever. This is not to say that vegans are at significant risk of a B12 deficiency because the history of vegetarian cultures does not suggest such a risk. Someone considering a strict vegetarian diet must understand, however, that most plants are poor sources of vitamin B12. If an adult beginning a strict vegetarian diet has normal stores of vitamin B12, it is not likely that that person will show any symptoms of a deficiency for many years. Nevertheless, fortified foods or vitamin supplements may be a prudent addition to a vegetarian diet.

The elderly may be at some small risk because it has been found that one-third of those over the age of sixty have diminished secretions of gastric acid. Without sufficient gastric acid, they cannot split the vitamin off from the protein complex in which it usually occurs in food. A very small percent of the elderly, perhaps as few as 1 percent, develop an inability to produce the intrinsic factor and are therefore less able to absorb vitamin B12. In addition, the efficiency of absorption is diminished in a pyridoxine (vitamin B6) deficiency, an iron deficiency, and in people with hypothyroidism.

Heavy drinkers are at some risk because alcohol depletes vitamin B12, and this warning applies to heavy smokers as well because tobacco decreases absorption. Anyone who takes megadoses of vitamin C or folic acid may develop deficiency symptoms because large quantities of vitamin C will destroy B12 and folacin can decrease blood levels of the vitamin.

Likely symptoms of a severe vitamin B12 deficiency are a sore tongue, general weakness, apathy, fatigue, back pains, tingling in the hands and feet, or some other nervous disorders such as difficulty in walking.

Technically, people recovering from gastrointestinal surgery or suffering from inflammation of the large or small intestine, such as ileitis, are at risk of a vitamin B12 deficiency because they may be unable to absorb the vitamin. In most cases, people on a diet devoid of the vitamin or those who cannot absorb the vitamin will develop a vitamin B12 deficiency slowly because the body carefully conserves the stores of B12 in the liver once it senses that they will not be replaced. In fact, it is thought that the liver is capable of storing up to a six-year supply of vitamin B12.

NOTE The likelihood of a vitamin B12 deficiency in a breast-fed infant is very slight. Reserves built up during the fetal life of the baby reduce the probability of a problem, unless the mother is a strict vegetarian. It should be noted that if the mother increases her intake of vitamin B12, an increase in B12 will be reflected in her breast milk from one to six days later.

STRATEGIES

FOOD SOURCES   There is no vitamin B12 in plant foods such as grains, vegetables, and fruits, and none in normal yeast, which is usually an outstanding source for other B-complex vitamins. The best sources of vitamin B12 are liver and organ meats, which is where the animal stores its vitamin B12. In addition, muscle meats, fish, eggs, and many milk products are good sources. The milk products that are only fair or poor sources are yogurt, evaporated milk, and butter. Pasteurizing milk depletes only about 10 percent of its vitamin B12, while 40 to 90 percent of the vitamin will be lost if the milk goes through an evaporation process.

FOOD PREPARATION More than half of the vitamin B12 found in food is in an unstable form and is easily destroyed by processing and other methods of food preparation. Beyond that, most of the vitamin that reaches your kitchen—about 70 percent—will not be lost by food preparation.

TOO MUCH VITAMIN B12 Vitamin B12 is considered nontoxic, which allows it to be used in significant quantities in the treatment of pernicious anemia and other deficiency disorders such as neurological disease or certain inherited metabolic errors. Otherwise, there is no point to taking extra vitamin B12 unless you have a known deficiency, which should be determined by your doctor.

DRUG INTERACTIONS Colchicine is a drug used to fight gout. It also destroys parts of the stomach lining, which creates a malabsorption of most nutrients including vitamin B12. As a result, this drug is usually taken for very short periods. If you suspect that you have a borderline deficiency in some vitamin, however, especially vitamin B12, it is advised that you take an all-purpose vitamin and mineral supplement.

Chloramphenicol (Chloromycetin), Erythromycin, and Sulfisoxazole and Sulfamethoxazole, antibiotics used to treat infections, increase the body's need for vitamin B12.

Cholestyramine, a drug that reduces cholesterol, will also reduce the absorption of B12, but it is very unlikely that the drug alone would produce a deficiency of any consequence. Another cholesterol reducer called Clofibrate (Atromid-S) may cause the malabsorption of vitamin B12 but, again, a vitamin deficiency would occur only after years of drug use.

Cycloserine (Seromycin), Para-Aminosalicylic Acid, and Isoniazid (INH and Rifamate) are antitubercular drugs that decrease the absorption of vitamin B12, making the vitamin less effective.

Oral contraceptives that contain estrogen and progestins may interfere with the effective absorption of vitamin B12. Long-term use of the anticancer drug Methotrexate (Folex and Mexate) could conceivably impair vitamin B12 absorption, and Phenobarbital, a powerful sedative, will also impair B12 absorption.

Penicillin inactivates vitamins B6 and B12, but a deficiency would occur only after long-term use. It has been reported that nitrous oxide, an anesthetic used in dental procedures, has produced a B12 deficiency in children who have had extensive dental work done.

People who have the need for potassium supplements to compensate for potassium depletion resulting from diuretics will find that these supplements will impair the absorption of vitamin B12. Again, a deficiency is not a likelihood unless the individual is already marginally deficient.

If you are taking one of these drugs, a suitable preventive measure would be to take a 3-microgram supplement. If you are concerned about a deficiency, see your physician.

BIOTIN

DESCRIPTION
As a coenzyme, biotin performs a critical role in the production and transformation of fatty acids, some amino acids and carbohydrates into energy. It is also vital to the production of glycogen which is stored in the liver and muscle tissue and is a necessary ingredient in the production of compounds that make up nucleic acids.

FOOD SOURCES
Excellent sources: liver, kidney (and other organ meats), egg yolk, nuts, cauliflower, legumes, and mushrooms

Good sources: oats, bulgur wheat, tuna, peanut butter, split peas, sunflower seeds, lentils, brown rice, cheese and butter

HIGH-RISK GROUPS FOR POSSIBLE DEFICIENCY
- anyone on a severe low-calorie diet
- people who eat large quantities of raw eggs
- heavy smokers

RECOMMENDED DOSAGE

GROUP	MCG	GROUP	MCG
Pregnant women	100–200	Children 7–10	120
Lactating women	100–200	Adults	100–200
Infants 0–0.6	35		
0.6–1	50		
Children 1–3	65		
4–6	85		

UPPER LIMITS FOR REGULAR DIETARY SUPPLEMENTAL USE

Children under 4 years of age: 225 mcg
Adults and children 4 or more years of age: 450 mcg
Pregnant or lactating women: 600 mcg

TOXIC LEVELS
Not known

BENEFITS

TREATING DEFICIENCY SYMPTOMS

BABIES:

- severe rash
- dry scaling scalp and face
- loss of hair
- lethargy
- depression

ADULTS:

- skin disorders

- smooth and pale tongue
- loss of appetite
- low-grade anemia
- lassitude and fatigue
- serious depression
- insomnia
- muscle pain

OTHER POSSIBLE BENEFITS

- eczema

UNPROVEN BENEFITS (UNRELATED TO DEFICIENCY SYMPTOMS)

- prevents baldness

TOXIC SYMPTOMS
There are no known symptoms for biotin toxicity.

DISCOVERY   As early as 1924 researchers suspected that they had "recognized" one of three dietary substances essential to the growth of microorganisms. They called this substance biosII. By 1940 biosII was identified as a vitamin, and it received the name biotin.

Two people in particular have received credit for their work on biotin. In 1940 Paul Gyorgy, a prominent biochemist, determined that biosII was, in fact, a vitamin, and he named it vitamin H. An American biochemist, Vincent Du Vigneaud, working at Cornell University Medical School, identified the same compound and by 1942 had deduced its complicated structure. Following Du Vigneaud's specifications, the chemists at Merck laboratories synthesized the compound the following year and learned that biosII, vitamin H, and biotin were all the same vitamin.

ROLE   Biotin, a white substance that contains sulfur in its molecule, as does thiamin, is considered an essential water-soluble vitamin. In the body biotin is bound to several enzymes by means of chemical union with a specific amino acid. In this combination, biotin assists in the transfer of carbon dioxide from the enzyme complex to other compounds. These reactions—called carboxylation reactions—play a part in the synthesis and oxidation of fatty acids and the oxidation of carbohydrates. Some of these reactions are closely involved with those of pantothenic acid.

Another function of biotin is promoting the synthesis of proteins, nicotinic acid, the production of energy from glucose, and the formation of some amino acids, glycogen, and nucleic acid.

PROBLEMS OF TOO LITTLE BIOTIN A naturally occurring deficiency of biotin in adults is not known. In fact, the dietary requirement for biotin is subject to question and possible revision because the amount known to be excreted in the urine and feces is greater than the known intake. What accounts for this difference is the fact the biotin is produced from microorganisms in the intestinal tract much like vitamin K. Part of the question surrounding the biotin requirement stems from the fact that we don't know how much, if any, of this biotin synthesized in the gut is absorbed and utilized by the body. Conceivably, all of the synthesized biotin could be excreted in the urine. Support for this theory stems from the fact that some farm animals, such as chickens and pigs, who synthesize biotin still develop a biotin deficiency if the vitamin is left out of their diet.

In studies designed to induce a deficiency in adults, the patients have exhibited symptoms similar to thiamin: skin disorders, loss of appetite, nausea, mental depression, and glossitis (smooth tongue).

WHO IS AT RISK Biotin deficiencies have been seen in adults and children who were fed intravenously (TPN or total parenteral nutrition). Because biotin had not been added to the TPN, both the infants and the adults developed symptoms similar to a biotin deficiency.

Two types of dermititis seen in some infants may be caused by a lack of biotin because when these infants were given larger doses of biotin (5 to 10 milligrams) the symptoms disappeared within hours. In some cases it is believed that the deficiency in these infants was caused by the absence at birth of certain enzymes that are essential for biotin absorption. Recent studies show that when pregnant women with a family history of this kind of deficiency were given high levels of biotin during their fifth month, their infants showed no evidence of biotin deficiency at the time of their birth.

NOTE A mother's breast milk, even if she has a normal diet and no inherited deficiency of biotin absorption, will still have only about one-tenth the amount of biotin of cow's milk. Women with a family history of this kind of deficiency should consult their pediatrician before electing to breast-feed.

Though some researchers believe that tobacco retards the absorption of biotin, a heavy smoker is not necessarily at risk of any biotin deficiency. But if he or she eats a severely restricted-calorie diet, a skin disorder might conceivably develop, traceable to a lack of biotin.

STRATEGIES

FOOD SOURCES Biotin is readily present in most foods. Most of it is bound to protein. The richest sources of biotin have been found in liver, kidney, peanut butter, egg yolks (not raw egg white), mushrooms, and yeast. To a lesser extent, wheat, fish, split peas (including lentils), sunflower seeds, some cheeses, and butter are satisfactory. But most other meats, fruits, and dairy products are only fair to poor sources of biotin.

The research concerning the availability of biotin from most food sources—namely its ability to be absorbed by the body—is still very new and inconclusive. For example, early results suggest that biotin in some cereals may be poorly absorbed.

FOOD PREPARATION Biotin is a highly durable water-soluble vitamin that is resistant to most processing procedures, long-term storage, and the heat of normal cooking.

DRUG INTERACTIONS There are no known drugs that will cause a potential biotin deficiency through short- or long-term use. Some nutritionists argue, however, that since broad-spectrum antibiotics and some sulfonamides (which are also antibiotics) destroy the intestinal bacteria necessary to the production of biotin in the body, a deficiency could develop when taking these drugs. This is a highly speculative concern since we don't know how much of this synthesized biotin is finally absorbed and used in the body.

FOLACIN (FOLIC ACID)

DESCRIPTION
Most of the biochemical roles of folacin are involved with blood formation. It plays a role in the metabolism and division of red blood cells and white blood cells. The iron-containing pigment found in red blood cells, called hemoglobin, require folic acid, as does the production of choline (see page 134). As a coenzyme, folic acid partners with vitamins B12 and C to break down and utilize proteins, and it is needed in the manufacture of nucleic acids, upon which all cellular growth and reproduction depend.

FOOD SOURCES
Excellent sources: wheat germ, brewer's yeast, broccoli, liver, and spinach
Good sources: green beans, asparagus, lima beans, lemons, orange juice, bananas, strawberries, and cantaloupe

HIGH-RISK GROUPS FOR POSSIBLE DEFICIENCY
- pregnant or breast-feeding women
- women who use oral contraceptives
- alcoholics
- people over 55 years
- people with wasting diseases
- people recovering from gastrointestinal surgery or severe burns
- people on a severe low-calorie diet
- people suffering from celiac disease
- people being fed intravenously
- infants who are neither breast-fed nor receiving fortified commercial formula
- heavy users of aspirin
- heavy users of vitamin C supplements

RECOMMENDED DOSAGE

GROUP	MCG	GROUP	MCG
Pregnant women	800	Children 7–10	300
Lactating women	1,200	Young women 11–22	400
Infants 0–0.6	30	Adult women 23+	400
0.6–1	45	Young men 11–18	400
Children 1–3	100	19–22	400
4–6	200	Adult men 23–50,	400
		51+	400

UPPER LIMITS FOR REGULAR DIETARY SUPPLEMENTAL USE

Children under 4 years of age: 300 mcg
Adults and children 4 or more years of age: 400 mcg
Pregnant or lactating women: 800–1,200 mcg

BENEFITS

TREATING DEFICIENCY SYMPTOMS
- paleness
- irritability
- fatigue
- sore red tongue
- diarrhea
- insomnia
- bleeding gums

GROSS DEFICIENCY
- mental confusion
- anemia (hemolytic or megaloblastic)

OTHER POSSIBLE BENEFITS
- toxemia of pregnancy (20 percent of pregnant women found to be deficient)

UNPROVEN BENEFITS (UNRELATED TO DEFICIENCY SYMPTOMS)

- treats depression
- prevents cervical cancer
- treats arthritis
- treats emphysema
- treats atherosclerosis
- prevents baldness

TOXIC SYMPTOMS

Folic acid is considered a nontoxic substance; however, excessive amounts may produce symptoms such as appetite loss, nausea, flatulence, and folacin crystals in the kidneys.

DISCOVERY   The history of science is filled with stories of researchers finding one thing when looking for another. Folacin, the second to last vitamin discovered, turned up when researchers were looking for the factor in beef liver that was responsible for curing or preventing pernicious anemia (see Vitamin B12, the last vitamin discovered, page 113). In fact, for many years these two vitamins were thought to be the same, and even today a deficiency of folacin is often mistaken for a vitamin B12 deficiency because they so closely resemble each other.

In 1930 a physician and biochemist named Lucy Wills working in Bombay, India, was concerned about the anemia she found in pregnant women patients. It was nutritional megaloblastic anemia, an anemia characterized by large (*mega*) red blood cells. By feeding monkeys a diet similar to that eaten by her patients, of polished rice and white bread, Dr. Wills was able to reproduce the same megaloblastic anemia.

When seeking a treatment for this disorder she was disappointed to learn that the megaloblastic anemia could not be corrected by the liver extract used to treat pernicious anemia (liver extract contains vitamin B12). However, when her patients were fed a yeast preparation, which reluctantly had been rejected as a cure for pernicious anemia, their symptoms improved. The discovery was that yeast contained what we know as folacin.

By 1945, following the formal discovery of folacin, it was determined that the vitamin cured megaloblastic anemia because it stimulated the growth of red blood cells and hemoglobin. Hemoglobin is the iron-containing pigment of red blood cells that carries oxygen from the lungs to the tissues. When the levels of red blood cells and hemoglobin fall, megaloblastic anemia results. Just as important, it was determined that folacin in some instances may reduce some of the symptoms of pernicious anemia, but it was not a cure because it could not correct the neurological symptoms. This finally ruled out the possibility that folacin was another form of vitamin B12.

The importance of these results was to establish that folacin and vitamin B12 were distinctly different vitamins with somewhat different capabilities and functions.

ROLE It could be said that the primary function of folic acid is to prevent megaloblastic anemia in humans. More specifically, once absorbed in the intestine, folacin is converted into a number of different coenzymes that are distributed throughout the body. Folacin, along with vitamin B12, is responsible for the production of essential components of red blood corpuscles. When adequate amounts of either vitamin are not available, red cell production drops and anemia develops.

Compounds dependent upon folacin coenzymes are needed for the synthesis of nucleic acids which are vital to all cell division and reproduction. Folacin coenzymes are also necessary for the manufacture of specific amino acids that are used in the formation of body proteins. Many of these reactions involving folic acid rely on other vitamins as well for their success, such as vitamins C, B6, and B12.

Perhaps its most important function is to transport single-carbon groups or units from one substance to another. These essential compounds are used in the makeup of the nucleic acids DNA and RNA, which are essential for the growth and reproduction of all body cells. The importance of these compounds rests in the fact that the new life of each cell is dependent upon DNA to carry its genetic code.

Folacin is needed to form the iron-containing protein hemoglobin, found in all red blood cells, and it plays a role in the formation of choline (see Choline, page 134).

PROBLEMS OF TOO LITTLE FOLACIN A lack of folic acid will result in a variety of symptoms such as red smooth tongue, gastrointestinal distress, and diarrhea. The principal symptom is a blood disorder called megaloblastic (or macrocytic) anemia in which there are fewer mature red blood cells present; they usually appear larger (megaloblasts) and contain less hemoglobin than is normal. As the deficiency continues, the immature red blood cells in the bone marrow simply fail to grow.

NOTE The cells on the surface of the tongue must be replaced continuously. When a folacin deficiency occurs, however, the surface of the tongue becomes smooth and painful because the folacin necessary for cell multiplication is not available.

WHO IS AT RISK It is estimated that approximately 10 percent of the American population have low stores of folacin. In adults, folic acid deficiencies appear to be limited generally to the elderly and women. Among this group some studies suggest that almost one-third have dietary intakes below the RDA recommendation and a minimum of one out of twenty has a severe deficiency.

Women have this vitamin deficiency for several reasons. The principal cause may be that oral contraceptives interfere with the absorption of the vitamin. Because of the increased demands of the fetus, pregnant women in their last trimester are at risk of megaloblastic anemia. The high incidence of folacin-deficiency megaloblastic anemia in lactating women points to the possibility that breast-feeding drains the mother's reserves. Because folic acid deficiency is the most prevalent nutritional problem among pregnant women, especially among women who have had many pregnancies, it is likely that many or most women begin lactation with seriously reduced reserves of folacin. For these reasons, and since screening for folacin blood levels is difficult and few laboratories conduct such tests, lactating women should assume a daily need of 1,200 micrograms.

About half of all people admitted to hospitals from low-income communities show some evidence of a folacin deficiency, which is a reflection of their poor diet. It is believed that 50 percent of alcoholics have a folacin deficiency because, in addition to a poor diet, problems of malabsorption, and liver damage, the alcohol they drink interferes with the absorption and metabolism of the vitamin.

In addition to those taking oral contraceptives, people who are taking certain prescriptive drugs such as anticonvulsants and some drugs used to treat tumors and malignancies (especially leukemia) risk a folic acid deficiency. (For a more complete list of drugs that can cause a folic acid deficiency, see Drug Interactions, page 128).

People suffering from celiac disease (a hereditary disorder involving an intolerance to gluten, a protein found in wheat and rye flours) are often unable to absorb a variety of nutrients, including many vitamins such as folic acid. Another malabsorption disorder called sprue, which is seen primarily in people from the Caribbean, India, and Southeast Asia, can cause a folic acid deficiency. Ironically, the disorder is also treated with folic acid, along with long-term antibiotics.

STRATEGIES

FOOD SOURCES   The information on folacin activity in foods for humans is relatively recent and incomplete because it has been difficult to measure the many different forms of folacin activity in animals. The ability for folacin to be absorbed depends, in part, on the presence of glutamic acid, which is needed to break the folacin away from the protein to which it is attached. Other factors of folacin absorption from food sources depend on the different types of binding involved, usually with a protein.

Nevertheless, it is well understood that the most concentrated source of folacin among foods is wheat germ. Close behind are liver, kidneys, yeast, and mushrooms. Most people don't eat much of these foods so their folacin needs must be provided by the fruits and vegetables they eat. Of the vegetables, asparagus, broccoli, green beans, lima beans, and spinach are the best choices, and the best fruit sources are oranges, followed by lemons, bananas, strawberries, and cantaloupe.

Poor sources of folacin are most meats, eggs, root vegetables (for example, potatoes and carrots), white flour, most desserts and processed milk, especially evaporated milk. On the other hand, cottage cheese is a relatively reliable source of folacin.

FOOD PREPARATION   Folacin is a water-soluble, heat-sensitive vitamin. This means that the processing and cooking of foods containing folacin may destroy as much as 50 to 90 percent of the vitamin. When high temperatures and a large volume of water are used, possibly all of the vitamin is lost. Cooking food in normal temperatures of approximately 110 degrees for about ten minutes will destroy 65 percent of the dietary folacin. The simple storing of fresh leafy vegetables, such as spinach, at room temperatures may cause them to lose up to 70 percent of their folacin activity. Generally speaking, microwave cooking will probably save far more folacin in foods than any other form of cooking.

SPECIAL ADVICE   Since folacin is water soluble and heat sensitive, it is best to cook vegetables in a pressure cooker. The next best method of preparation is steaming. If you must boil your vegetables, use as little water as possible. Also, cooking folacin-rich foods in copper utensils will accelerate the destruction of the vitamin.

DRUG INTERACTIONS   Chronic use of aspirin will increase the likelihood of a folacin deficiency because it increases the loss of folacin in the urine. Busulfan (Myleran), an anticancer agent that prevents the formation of healthy and unhealthy cells, also impairs the absorption of nutrients, including folic acid, through the lining of the intestine.

Pyrimethamine (Daraprim and Fansidar) and Trimethoprim are used in the treatment of malaria. They are also potent antagonists since they prevent folacin from being converted into its active form. Taken over an extended period they could conceivably produce a deficiency. Triamterene is another drug that prevents the vitamin from being converted into its active form.

Cholestyramine (Questran) and Colestipol Hydrochloride (Colestid) lower blood cholesterol levels, but they also create potential absorption problems for folic acid.

Cycloserine (Seromycin), Para-Aminosalicylic Acid, and Isoniazid (INH and Rifamate) are antitubercular drugs that impair the absorption of folic acid and make the vitamin less effective.

Chloramphenicol, Neomycin, Erythromycin, Sulfisoxazole, Sulfamethoxazole, and Tetracycline are all antibiotics used to treat infections that also increase the body's need for folic acid.

Oral contraceptives that contain estrogen and progestins will increase the excretion of folic acid. Long-term use of the anticancer drug Methotrexate (Folex and Mexate) will impair folic acid absorption, as will Phenobarbital, a powerful sedative.

Penicillin decreases the body's ability to use folacin. People who take corticosteroids, drugs that accelerate the reactions in the body, will also decrease the effect of folic acid.

Phenytoin (Dilantin) and Primidone (Mysoline), an anti-epileptic drug, can decrease the absorption of folacin in the body.

PANTOTHENIC ACID

DESCRIPTION

Pantothenic acid plays a significant role in the metabolism of cells. As a coenzyme this water-soluble vitamin participates in the metabolism of carbohydrates, proteins, and fats, and in the metabolism of riboflavin (vitamin B2). It is essential in the synthesis of cholesterol and fatty acids and in the maintenance of a healthy digestive tract. It also aids in the formation of hormones and nerve-regulating substances.

FOOD SOURCES

Excellent sources: yeast, egg yolks, beef liver, lamb kidneys, wheat bran and wheat germ, sunflower seeds, peanuts, peas, and watermelon
Good sources: poultry (dark meat), milk, sardines, salmon, chick-peas, broccoli, avocados, whole wheat bread, and blue cheese

HIGH-RISK GROUPS FOR POSSIBLE DEFICIENCY

- heavy users of alcohol
- people recovering from gastrointestinal surgery or severe burns
- people suffering from a wasting disease
- people on severe low-calorie diets
- heavy smokers
- people involved in vigorous physical activities
- pregnant or breast-feeding women

RECOMMENDED DOSAGE

GROUP	MG	GROUP	MG
Pregnant women	7–10	Young women 11–14	4–7
Lactating women	7–10	15–18	4–7
Infants 0–.6	2	19–22	4–7
.6–1	3	Adult women 23–50	5–10
Children 1–3	3	51+	5–10
4–6	3–4	Young men 11–14	5–10
7–10	4–5	15–18	5–10
		19–22	5–10
		Adult men 23–50	5–10
		51+	5–10

UPPER LIMITS FOR REGULAR DIETARY SUPPLEMENTAL USE

Children under 4 years of age: 7.5 mg
Adults and children 4 or more years of age: 15 mg
Pregnant or lactating women: 20 mg

BENEFITS

TREATING DEFICIENCY SYMPTOMS

A severe lack of pantothenic acid would impair the health of the cells in many tissues, but under natural conditions no known deficiency of pantothenic acid has been seen. In experiments with volunteers, using a purified diet and specific drugs that are antagonistic to the vitamin, the following deficiency symptoms were observed:

- fatigue
- headaches
- sleep disorders
- personality changes
- nausea
- abdominal distress
- numbness and tingling in the extremities
- muscle cramps
- difficulty in walking and impaired coordination

POSSIBLE BENEFITS

- treating paralysis of the gastrointestinal tract after surgery (reducing the accumulation of gas that can be the cause of severe abdominal pain)

UNPROVEN BENEFITS (UNRELATED TO DEFICIENCY SYMPTOMS)

- treats baldness
- aids in the treatment of epilepsy and multiple sclerosis
- treats symptoms of arthritis and gout
- provides protection against allergies

TOXIC SYMPTOMS

Diarrhea and water retention (with megadoses of more than 10,000 milligrams).

DISCOVERY Pantothenic acid was the third of the B-complex family of vitamins to be isolated. Initially called vitamin B5, pantothenic acid was given its present name in 1933 by the American biochemist R. J. Williams who finally isolated the vitamin after fifteen years of research at Oregon State University.

When pantothenic acid was first isolated, it was the unknown factor necessary to the growth of yeast. In subsequent experiments with test animals, it was found to be effective in the cure or prevention of skin disorders in chicks and of the graying of hair in rats. Eventually it was learned that the vitamin was part of the vitamin B complex needed by all higher organisms. Its chemical structure was determined by 1940.

ROLE Testing with animals has revealed a number of this vitamin's functions. The most dramatic evidence found was when test animals, fed a diet deficient in pantothenic acid, developed enlarged adrenal glands that caused hemorrhaging and, eventually, slowed growth.

How pantothenic acid is involved in adrenal activity became apparent only after it was learned that the vitamin was a part of coenzyme A because the task of the coenzyme is to assist in making cortisone and two other related hormones in the adrenal glands. Without these hormones, which are critical to most regulatory functions, the body would eventually die.

In its partnership with coenzyme A, pantothenic acid is necessary to the synthesis, breakdown, and release of energy from fats, proteins, and carbohydrates, the maintenance of blood-sugar levels, and an effective defense against infection. It also aids in the production of a substance called acetylcholine, which plays an important role in the transmission of nerve impulses in the body.

In the performance of all its various roles, the vitamin has a complicated and interdependent relationship with numerous other nutrients. For example, pantothenic acid relies on other coenzymes that contain vitamins, such as thiamin (B1), riboflavin (B2), niacin (B3), pyridoxine (B6), and biotin. It also needs the cooperation of specific minerals such as phosphorus, sulfur, magnesium, and manganese.

Because of its many different essential metabolic roles, pantothenic acid has earned the reputation as the one vitamin that "sits at the crossroads of metabolism."

PROBLEMS OF TOO LITTLE A deficiency of pantothenic acid is so uncommon in this country that much of what we know about significant deficiency symptoms is a result of experiments with test animals.

In an effort to learn about the various functions of the vitamin, test animals were fed diets that had been heated so as to destroy the vitamin. (A pantothenic acid deficiency does not occur naturally in animals or humans.) Chicks fed this deficient diet grew poorly and developed a characteristic dermatitis on their break and around their eyes. In other test animals the deficiency affected other tissues, causing poor overall growth and impairing reproduction. When the hair of tested rats, monkeys, and dogs turned gray, their hair color could be restored simply by adding the vitamin to their diet. (This is not an indication that pantothenic acid has any capability of retarding or eliminating the graying of human hair.)

Despite the fact that a case of pantothenic acid deficiency is relatively rare, doctors have seen many cases in which low intakes of the vitamin have slowed the entire metabolic process of the patient, resulting principally in a condition of general fatigue. Some people have also experienced insomnia and mild depression with extremely low intakes of the vitamin. Poor dietary intakes have also resulted in a lowered resistance to infection, while increased intakes have improved resistance to stress.

WHO IS AT RISK   A normal diet provides all the pantothenic acid most people need, making deficiencies relatively rare. However, anyone with a deficient diet, whether it is a severe low-calorie diet or a long history of poor eating habits, is exposed to an increased risk of developing some possible pantothenic acid deficiency symptoms. The active alcoholic or heavy drinker is frequently someone whose eating habits have produced a variety of vitamin and mineral deficiencies, including pantothenic acid. Some studies show that tobacco decreases the absorption of pantothenic acid, too.

People who have difficulty absorbing nutrients, especially people recovering from gastrointestinal surgery or severe burns, may exhibit some signs. The demands of a pregnancy or periods of breast-feeding may result in the need for more pantothenic acid.

NOTE   As in the case of vitamins A and C, cow's milk provides more pantothenic acid than does human milk.

STRATEGIES

FOOD SOURCES   Because pantothenic acid is a part of all living matter, it appears in virtually all natural foods, especially yeast (in which it was first found), liver, eggs, wheat germ, peanuts, and peas. Sweet potatoes, mushrooms, meats, poultry, milk, and broccoli are also good sources, but most vegetables and fruits are relatively disappointing.

Needless to say, most refined foods are also relatively poor. Absolutely no pantothenic acid is found in salad oils, shortening, and sugar.

FOOD PREPARATION   Pantothenic acid is relatively stable in moist heat (steaming), but in high dry heat much of the pantothenic acid can be destroyed. Foods that are processed in dry heat, for example, are relatively poor sources of pantothenic acid. Canned foods for animals lose from 20 to 35 percent of their pantothenic acid content. Canned vegetables lose from 50 to 80 percent. Though you have no control over the refining of wheat, it is estimated that about 50 percent is lost in the process.

TOO MUCH   There is no known toxic level for the use of pantothenic acid.

DRUG INTERACTIONS   There are no known drugs that will cause a potential pantothenic acid deficiency through short- or long-term use.

OTHER VITAMINLIKE SUBSTANCES

Foods contain other vitaminlike substances that have many of the characteristics of vitamins but are not formally considered vitamins because they fail to meet all the criteria to be classified as vitamins. They appear to have some essential role in the healthy functioning of the body, but it is not clear whether they are needed in our diet because the body produces the quantities it needs. Many of them are widely distributed throughout our foods, and some are found in greater quantities in our body than are vitamins.

The vitaminlike substances we will discuss are choline, inositol, and carnitine. Much of the newest research has been devoted to uncovering the various functions of these substances; in one instance, carnitine was discovered to be helpful in saving the lives of children born with genetically induced vitaminlike deficiencies.

It is conceivable that in time research will prove one or more of these substances deserving of classification as a vitamin. Until that time arrives, there is little or no evidence that adults require any supplementation of these vitaminlike substances in their diets.

NOTE Some nutritionists consider the amino acid *taurine* a vitaminlike substance because it serves as a building block of proteins. Another argument regarding the importance of taurine to humans is that relatively high amounts in maternal breast milk suggest that it is important to the development process, especially for brain development. There is no evidence, however, that there is a dietary need for taurine.

CHOLINE

DESCRIPTION

Despite the claim of some nutritionists that choline is considered one of the B-complex vitamins, it is not. Formally, it is considered a vitamin only for some animals. Choline does appear to be vital to the functioning of a healthy nervous system, however, and it is essential for the metabolism of other lipids, which are fats or fatlike substances.

FOOD SOURCES
Excellent sources: egg yolks, beef liver, whole grains, wheat germ, and most meats
Good sources: garbanzo beans, soybeans, split peas, lentils, green beans, and fish

HIGH-RISK GROUPS FOR POSSIBLE DEFICIENCY
Generally speaking, no one group is considered a risk for a choline deficiency. Since infants are as yet unable to synthesize choline, however, it is added to their formula. Also, possibly alcoholics may need it to prevent liver damage.

SAFE LEVELS
12 milligrams daily

BENEFITS
TREATING DEFICIENCY SYMPTOMS
None are known.

OTHER POSSIBLE BENEFITS
Protects against cirrhosis of the liver.

UNPROVEN BENEFITS (UNRELATED TO DEFICIENCY SYMPTOMS)
- treats Alzheimer's disease
- lowers blood cholesterol levels
- protects against the arterial damage of hypertension
- treats nephritis
- prevents glaucoma

TOXIC SYMPTOMS
None are known for humans.

DISCOVERY Choline was discovered as early as 1862 by a German chemist who seemingly isolated the substance from bile. Its animal vitamin properties went undiscovered, however, until it was determined through exhaustive tests in the 1940s that the growth of rats depended on choline.

About ten years earlier, Canadian researchers learned that lecithin, a fatty substance called a phospholipid that contained choline in its molecule, was effective in preventing fatty livers in dogs. By breaking out all the various components of lecithin, they were able to determine that the choline in the lecithin was responsible for preventing or curing fatty livers in a variety of test animals that were fed low-protein, high-fat, and high-cholesterol diets. In 1942 further experiments finally confirmed the vitaminlike nature and properties of choline.

ROLE   Choline has a number of important functions in the body. Unlike most vitamins, it does not catalyze any reactions, nor is it a part of a coenzyme, but as a constituent part of lecithin, a phospholipid, it aids in the transportation of fat throughout the body. As part of another phospholipid called a sphingomyelin, it is important for nerve cell membranes, too.

PROBLEMS OF TOO LITTLE CHOLINE   There is little documented evidence of choline deficiency in humans because it is rarely ever seen. This is partly explained by the fact that the body appears capable of producing all the choline it needs, except in the case of infants. Though the requirement for choline in infants is basically unknown, a standard has been established for infant formulas by the American Academy of Pediatrics because a deficiency of choline could conceivably place an infant at risk of liver and kidney damage.

Generally, what we know about choline deficiency symptoms stems from animal tests in which rats, guinea pigs, pigs, monkeys, dogs, and calves were fed diets with insufficient choline. All of the animals developed fatty livers in four to six weeks. When the deficiency continued, some of the animals eventually developed impaired cardiovascular systems and bleeding of the liver and heart muscle.

A need for choline may occur among alcoholics because excessive fat will build up in their livers, as it will in people on a severe low-protein diet, and in children suffering from kwashiorkor, a disease resulting from a protein deficiency.

Problems of disorientation and other neurological disorders have been associated with deficiencies in various nutrient factors, especially vitamins B1, B3, and B6. It appears that a gross deficiency of choline will cause similar problems because it will interfere with the production of a neurotransmitter called acetylcholine.

WHO IS AT RISK   No one is naturally at risk of a choline deficiency.

STRATEGIES

FOOD SOURCES   Choline is widely distributed in food and is present in large amounts in foods that contain fat, specifically foods that contain phospholipids (fatty substances that contain phosphorus). Eggs are a good source of phospholipids, while fruits and vegetables contain virtually none. The average American diet provides from 500 to 900 milligrams daily, which appears to be all the body requires.

With the additional supplement from the body's synthesis of choline, there seems to be no call for additional intakes.

FOOD PREPARATION   Choline is water soluble and relatively stable. It exists in foods in phospholipids and crystalline salts. It is heat resistant and is not destroyed even when stored over long periods.

DRUG INTERACTIONS Anyone taking excessive amounts of nicotinic acid (nicotinamide or vitamin B3) may be at some mild risk of a deficiency because this vitamin decreases choline effectiveness.

INOSITOL

DESCRIPTION
Inositol, a vitaminlike substance often grouped among the B-complex vitamins, is associated with the production of lecithin in the body. Although it is thought to be associated with cell growth in the liver and bone marrow, and perhaps prevents fatty livers, its specific role in human nutrition is still unclear.

FOOD SOURCES
Good sources: brewer's yeast, citrus fruits (except lemons), calf's liver, pork, veal, milk, vegetables, nuts and whole-grain cereals

HIGH-RISK GROUPS FOR POSSIBLE DEFICIENCY
Most of the higher animals and humans appear capable of synthesizing all the inositol they need; therefor there is no established dietary levels.

RECOMMENDED DOSAGE
In 1982 the Food and Drug Administration established a minimum level of 4 milligrams for infant formu

TOXIC LEVELS
Not established.

BENEFITS
TREATING DEFICIENCY SYMPTOMS
Not established.

UNPROVEN BENEFITS (UNRELATED TO DEFICIENCY SYMPTOMS)
- controls blood cholesterol levels and hypertension
- prevents baldness
- prevents asthma
- eases constipation
- acts as a sedative

TOXIC SYMPTOMS
None known in humans.

DISCOVERY Inositol, which is a group name for a number of carbon compounds closely related to glucose, was first recognized in 1928 as an essential growth factor for certain yeasts and as a cure for loss of hair in mice. Later research pointed to their importance in the growth of some bacteria, some lower organisms, and some fish (possibly sharks).

Inositol appears under other forms and other names. In addition to being called muscle sugar and mesoinositol, in its most active form— myoinositol—it is found in virtually all plants and animal tissues. In animal cells it occurs as a phospholipid, a fatty substance that contains phosphorus. Choline is another phospholipid.

ROLE The biological significance of inositol for humans has not been established, but it is widely distributed in the brain, heart, and skeletal muscle.

PROBLEMS OF TOO LITTLE INOSITOL The biological need for inositol in human nutrition is not known, but deficiency symptoms have been seen in experimental animals. In addition to a diet that offers about one gram per day, humans are capable of synthesizing enough inositol, with the aid of glucose, to meet most needs.

CARNITINE

DESCRIPTION
Carnitine is a vital coenzyme in animal tissue and essential to the transportation of long-chain fatty acids into the cell where it is metabolized.

FOOD SOURCES
Good sources: dark red meat and most dairy products

HIGH-RISK GROUPS FOR POSSIBLE DEFICIENCY
Most of the higher animals and humans appear capable of synthesizing all the carnitine they need.

RECOMMENDED DOSAGE
In 1982 the Food and Drug Administration established a minimum level of 4 milligrams for infant formula.

TOXIC LEVELS
Not established.

BENEFITS
TREATING DEFICIENCY SYMPTOMS
Not established.

UNPROVEN BENEFITS (UNRELATED TO DEFICIENCY SYMPTOMS)
Not established.

TOXIC SYMPTOMS
None known in humans.

DISCOVERY   A human deficiency in carnitine was first recognized in 1973, primarily in people who were unable to synthesize the substance. Prior to this discovery carnitine was known only as an essential growth factor for insects. It was once called vitamin Bt.

ROLE   The biological significance of carnitine in some respects resembles choline and inositol in that it is a vital coenzyme in animal tissue and central to fat metabolism in their cells. Its chemical structure is similar to choline, but it cannot prevent or treat a choline deficiency. Carnitine is widely distributed in most animal foods.

PROBLEMS OF TOO LITTLE CARNITINE
The requirements for carnitine are not known, but as humans are usually able to synthesize enough for their own needs, deficiencies are rare.

WHO IS AT RISK   No one is naturally at risk for a carnitine deficiency. Some newborn infants are unable to produce sufficient carnitine to maintain appropriate blood levels, however, and in these instances the infants should be breast-fed. When these infants are bottle-fed, they exhibit an inability to use fatty acids, which results in unregulated body heat and elevated blood lipids. In the view of many physicians, the higher carnitine content of breast milk compared to cow's milk is another argument for the choice of breast milk in the early life of an infant.

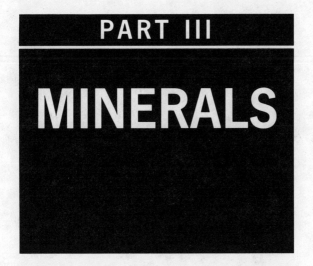

PART III

MINERALS

There are about ninety different chemical elements in nature, and at least twenty-one of them are present in our bodies. Most of them have proven to be important, if not essential, to human nutrition, while some few of them may have no discernable role—but researchers suspect they could be important.

The measure of their usefulness or indispensability is whether they perform a function that affects growth or overall health. This means that if an essential element is added to our diet, there should be an improvement in our functioning, and if the element is removed, there should be some sign of a deficiency. This is the basic test for a nutrient in most animal studies.

We will discuss twenty-four elements, of which twenty-one are considered essential to human nutrition. We have included at least three nonessential elements because studies involving their nutritional possibilities have sparked interest in some researchers regarding their future consideration as "essential" micronutrients.

Though these elements make up about only 5 percent of our overall weight, they are critical to our good health. They are key components of our bones, teeth, soft tissue, muscle, blood, and nerve cells; they are also central to good digestion and metabolism, proper muscle response, and the effective operation of our nervous system. Without them we could not maintain our delicate internal water balances or ensure that our bodily fluids, including our blood supply, do not become too acidic or alkaline. Minerals also work to draw chemical substances in and out of the cells and aid in the creation of antibodies.

In short, life as we know it could not exist without them.

HOW THEY ARE GROUPED The nutritional minerals present in our bodies are divided into two groups. This arrangement has nothing to do with their function. Rather, they are divided as macronutrients or micronutrients (sometimes referred to as trace elements) on the basis of the quantity found in our bodies.

The macrominerals represent those elements that are found in our body and food supply in significant amounts. They are calcium, phosphorus, magnesium, potassium, sodium, sulfur, and chloride. Microminerals are those elements that are present in small amounts but are also essential to a healthy life. These so-called trace elements are iron, copper, iodine, zinc, fluoride, chromium, manganese, molybdenum, nickel, cobalt, arsenic, vanadium, silicon, and selenium. (The importance of tin, lead, and boron has not been as well demonstrated as the others in human studies, but deficiencies of these elements, in some experimental animals, suggest that they, too, may one day be viewed as essential to good human nutrition.)

Vitamins get a lot of attention as necessary to a good diet, yet it is the inorganic minerals that demonstrate, perhaps more dramatically, the importance of a varied and balanced diet. The minerals we need are not present in all foods, and some are found only in limited amounts. Iodine, which is needed for the production of thyroid hormones that control the rate at which the cells in the body work, is found in minute amounts primarily in cheese, eggs, kelp, meat, milk, seafood, and some vegetables. At one time it was thought there was so little iodine in the American diet that it had to be added to common table salt (iodized) to ensure proper levels for everyone.

Minerals and vitamins are not strangers to each other. As coworkers they help one another get absorbed into the body. Calcium, for example, is more effectively absorbed when taken with foods rich in vitamins A and C; and vitamin D makes it possible for the calcium to be retained. Furthermore, vitamin C helps iron and magnesium be absorbed, while vitamin A performs the same task for zinc and phosphorus.

In addition to cooperation, balance is another principle of our physiological functions. Too much of a good thing may add up to be a bad thing. For example, minerals affect each other: the more you take of one, the greater the effect on others. In the case of zinc, too much (particularly taken as a supplement) can create a deficiency of copper, a mineral that helps form red blood cells. Another example is phosphorus which, if taken in excessive quantities, may interfere with our ability to use calcium.

MINERAL DEFICIENCIES   A mineral deficiency can occur when there is too little of the mineral or too much of another in our diet, or too much of the mineral is excreted or not enough is absorbed. Mineral deficiencies are not common; in fact, with a few exceptions they are usually quite rare. When a deficiency occurs, however, it can be very troublesome, even life-threatening.

Of the macronutrients, dietary calcium is the only one of which many people are deficient. It is estimated, for example, that one out of every four postmenopausal women suffers from a weakening of the bones caused, in part, by a deficiency of calcium. Since 98 percent of the calcium is stored in the bones, a significant calcium deficiency will weaken the bones, making them soft. If the deficiency continues, they can become so brittle that they will fracture and break.

Deficiencies are relatively unknown among the trace minerals, with the exception of iron. Iron, which is essential to the blood's oxygen-carrying capacity, is the most common nutritional deficiency in this country, especially in women. An iron shortage results in anemia, signaled by such symptoms as tiredness and general feelings of malaise, irritability, and breathlessness.

Unlike vitamins, the macronutrients and micronutrients found in our food are not destroyed or easily lost by cooking, improper storage, or even aging of our food. Another difference between minerals and vitamins, albeit small, is their source. Our diet remains our principal source for most vitamins, whereas it is our *only* source for *ALL* minerals.

The foods of animal origin contain higher concentrations of minerals, and the minerals are more readily absorbed than those found in plants. Meats, especially liver, kidney, and other organ meats, are excellent choices for many minerals. Whole grains are generally believed to contain many essential minerals, especially in the outer layers and the germ. Unfortunately, milling removes some of the minerals, and the fiber in the husk of grains tends to impair the absorption of the minerals.

TOXICITY At various levels all elements, including minerals, can become toxic in the body. While the lack of an element can result in harmful deficiency symptoms, and in some cases it could be fatal, an excessive amount of that same element could become poisonous and life-threatening. This is true of both macronutrients and micronutrients.

Another problem involving a high intake of a mineral is malabsorption. Ingesting large quantities of one mineral can block another from being properly absorbed. The acceptable level of need will vary from element to element, but with the exception of iron supplements, an all-purpose daily supplement should provide all the minerals a healthy person requires.

MINERAL SUPPLEMENTS More and more information is becoming available about the role of minerals in our diets. In fact, much of recent nutrition research has been devoted to the possible nutritional function of many trace elements. All this attention on minerals has occasioned a significant increase in the sales of mineral supplements in the form of pills and capsules. In most cases self-medication with mineral supplements is a risky business, and the hazards of doing so are well documented.

Minerals function in concert with each other, and they affect each other as well. Because of these complex interrelationships, seldom does a single uncomplicated deficiency exist under normal conditions. In other words, to treat one suspected mineral deficiency may create problems with others.

With the exception of calcium, iron, and iodine (in the form of iodized salt), which are the only mineral elements the FDA believes are justified as dietary supplements, it is generally unwise to take mineral supplements without a doctor's supervision. What you see as a need for mineral supplements is what your physician should see as well.

In most cases a well-balanced diet provides more than enough minerals for most healthy people. If you are on a low-calorie diet and are worried about your mineral intake, it is recommended that you add those foods to your diet that contain the minerals in question. Many foods rich in minerals are also low in calories, such as vegetables, seafood, poultry, and eggs.

CALCIUM

DESCRIPTION

Calcium is important to the formation of rigid and firm bones and teeth. It also plays a role in lactation, activating enzymes, and in the function of muscles, nerves, and cell tissue. To a lesser extent it is involved in blood coagulation and establishing the acid-base balance of the blood.

FOOD SOURCES

Excellent sources: skim milk, cottage cheese, low-fat yogurt, egg yolk, sardines, and canned salmon
Good sources: whole milk, cream and hard cheeses, almonds, brewer's yeast, oysters, collard and mustard greens, kelp, soybean curd, walnuts, and watercress

HIGH-RISK GROUPS FOR POSSIBLE DEFICIENCY

- postmenopausal women
- individuals with osteoporosis in immediate family
- fair-skinned women who are small and thin
- people with lactose intolerance
- long-term low-calorie dieters
- heavy smokers
- alcoholics
- people homebound and bedridden
- people who take the antibiotic Tetracycline or Erythromycin
- people who take Methotrexate (Folex and Mexate), a cancer drug
- people who take Isoniazid ("INH and Rifamate) or Cycloserine (Seromycin), antitubercular drugs
- people who regularly use potassium-based saline cathartics, diphenylmethane cathartics, or mineral oil as laxatives
- people who take antacids that contain magnesium hydroxide
- people who take the diuretics Ethacrynic Acid and Sodium Ethacrynate, Furosemide, Spironolactone, Thiazides, and mercurial diuretics (Diamox, Daranide, and Neptazane)
- people who take corticosteroids

RECOMMENDED DOSAGE

GROUP	MG	GROUP	MG
Pregnant women	1,200	Children 7–10	800
Lactating women	1,200	Young women 11–14	1200
Infants .0–.6	360	15–18	1200
.6–1.0	540	19–22	1200
Children 1–3	800	Young men 11–14	1200
4–6	800	15–18	1200
		19–22	1200
		Adults 23–50	800

UPPER LIMITS OF REGULAR DIETARY SUPPLEMENTAL USE

Children under 4 years of age: 1,200 mg
Adults and children over 4 years of age: 1,500 mg
Pregnant or lactating women: 2,000 mg

DEFICIENCY SYMPTOMS

- nervousness
- muscle cramps
- numbness and tingling in arms and legs
- brittle bones
- dental decay
- bleeding gums

OTHER POSSIBLE BENEFITS

- treatment of hypertension (but not with the use of supplements)

UNPROVEN BENEFITS (UNRELATED TO DEFICIENCY SYMPTOMS)

- treatment of nephritis
- treats allergies
- treats diabetes
- acts as a tranquilizer and prevents insomnia
- treats celiac disease
- used in the treatment of Meniere's disease

TOXIC SYMPTOMS

Drowsiness, extreme lethargy.

DISCOVERY   Calcium is a silver-white metallic element that, among other things, is a major component of limestone and human bones. A 160-pound man carries approximately 3 pounds of calcium (a woman slightly less), and 98 percent of it is found in the bones, the rest in teeth and soft tissue. Despite the fact that it has been used for ages as a component of lime, it was not identified as a separate mineral until the early nineteenth century.

In 1808 the English chemist Sir Humphry Davy, who won fame with his experiments on electricity, discovered that through an electrical charge he could isolate a number of minerals, including calcium. This was the first time calcium was so identified; however, any understanding regarding its role in nutrition was to wait for another hundred years. (Calcium derives from the Latin *calx* which means chalk, of which calcium is a major part.)

Near the close of World War I chemists were studying the effects of certain minerals on the growth of rats. They learned that rats could handle shortages of magnesium, potassium, sodium, and chlorine, but they could not adapt to a shortage of phosphorus and calcium. These two minerals seemed essential to normal growth.

An American chemist named Henry Clapp Sherman furthered the work of these experiments and eventually demonstrated that calcium and phosphorus were required for proper growth in children. (He also worked with the problem of rickets.) Elmer McCollum, whose work on vitamins A and D was so important to the history of nutrition (see Vitamin A, page 56, and Vitamin D, page 63), also determined that a deficiency of calcium would produce tetany (see Problems of Too Little Calcium).

ROLE While calcium is best known as the principal element for building strong bones and teeth, the tiny proportion of calcium that is used for other tasks is critical to a healthy life. It promotes good metabolism by activating several enzymes and is instrumental in muscle growth and muscle contraction. As an ion (an electrically charged atom) calcium is involved in the clotting of blood. On its own, calcium only marginally affects the acid and alkaline balance of the blood; but when taken in the form of calcium bicarbonate supplement, it will significantly affect the pH of the blood. The bicarbonate in the compound, which is a salt, "buffers" the blood, which means it tends to preserve its proper hydrogen-ion concentration by neutralizing its acids and bases.

ACID-BASE BALANCE The pH, or acid base balance, of a solution refers to the concentration of the hydrogen ion (+) of a solution. If the solution is measured as a 7, it means the solution is considered neutral because the acids (+) and bases (−) in the solution are the same. A solution with a pH of 0 to 6.9 is acidic, and one that is 7.1 to 14 is considered alkaline (or basic). In other words, an acid solution has more hydrogen ions than a neutral solution, and an alkaline solution contains fewer hydrogen ions than a neutral solution.

The importance of an acid-base balance is that many biological reactions within the cell can occur only when the pH is within a very narrow range. The ions or electrical charges come from the minerals found in the food we eat. Chlorine, sulfur, and phosphorus form acids when dissolved in water, and base-forming minerals are calcium, potassium, sodium, and magnesium.

The acid-forming elements tend to appear in foods containing protein, such as meat, eggs, and cereals. Alkaline or base-forming elements are found in greater quantity in fruits, vegetables, and nuts.

Calcium is essential to a healthy heart. Insufficient calcium may actually slow the contractions of the heart muscle and cause them to become irregular. For this reason heart patients suffering from congestive heart failure, which occurs when the heart does not pump blood fast enough, are given calcium as part of their therapy. Calcium also helps in the stimulation of nerves, which is essential to its transmission function.

In order for nutrients to pass in and out of tissue cells, calcium must be present to maintain the permeability of the cell walls. Lactating mothers would be unable to nurse their babies if it were not for calcium. Finally, as part of a common task shared by many minerals, calcium assists other minerals and vitamin B12 in their absorption. In this case calcium benefits iron, magnesium, and phosphorus absorption.

PROBLEMS OF TOO LITTLE CALCIUM Unfortunately, calcium deficiencies are not uncommon. One of the first signs of a calcium deficiency is a nervous affliction called tetany (not to be confused with tetanus), which is characterized by muscle cramps and numbness and tingling in the arms and legs. Peridontal disease and poor teeth formation or teeth decay may be a sign of a longer-term calcium deficiency. Recent studies indicate that some people with high blood pressure may also have low or poor blood calcium levels.

Deficiencies occur when the level of calcium that is dissolved and circulating in the blood system falls to a point that the body must begin to liberate whatever amount it needs from the bones where calcium is stored. If this bone calcium loss continues for four or five years without the mineral being replaced, the bones would weaken, become soft, and eventually be more susceptible to fractures. This uniform and steady loss of bone calcium is called *osteomalacia,* a condition that may be reversed if calcium levels are returned to normal. Signs of osteomalacia are bone pain in the back, thighs, shoulders, or ribs. Other symptoms are dental caries, rickets, difficulty in walking, a weakness in the muscles of the legs, and in some rare instances, excessive bleeding.

A longer period of calcium deficiency can contribute to a sudden loss of calcium from the bones. This condition is called *osteoporosis,* and it has been generally considered irreversible. Some studies have shown, however, that exercise, even in elderly women, can contribute to a gain of bone growth, but the benefit of increased dietary calcium at this stage may only serve to prevent the condition from getting worse.

In an advanced case of osteoporosis, bones grow brittle and break easily. The first symptoms are similar to osteomalacia; backache, poor posture, and periodontal disease.

It is very difficult for most people to distinguish between the early symptoms of osteomalacia and osteoporosis. It is best to look at your diet and determine whether you consume adequate calcium. If you almost never eat foods high in calcium (see table on page 244) and haven't done so for years, then these symptoms probably point to osteomalacia because this disease is caused by long-term calcium deficiencies. On the other hand, if your diet regularly contains calcium-rich foods or if you have been taking calcium supplements, these same symptoms would more likely suggest osteoporosis because this disease can be the result of factors other than a calcium deficiency.

It is believed by some experts that only 13 percent of the hip fractures in this country, a common sign of osteoporosis, are due to low calcium intake per se. Studies indicate, in fact, that osteoporosis, which affects 24 million Americans, is caused by at least two factors other than poor calcium intake. Dr. Steven R. Cummings of the University of California School of Medicine in San Francisco attributes 10 to 20 percent of hip fractures to cigarette smoking. Besides the direct effect of smoking in depleting calcium, Cummings believes that these numbers reflect, in part, the relative deficiency of estrogen (the female sex hormone) in women who smoke. Researchers believe the absence of estrogen is the new key to the bone loss disease of osteoporosis.

In advanced cases of osteoporosis, fractures of the hip, vertebrae, and wrist can occur frequently, sometimes spontaneously. But the most dramatic symptom of osteoporosis is a gradual loss of height. We notice this phenomenon especially in the elderly. The loss of height occurs when the bones in the spinal vertebrae are crushed and worn down because they are too weak to bear the weight of the body. The breakdown is most noticeable at the ends of the bone and in those areas subject to great pressure. Consequently, the frame is literally shortened. Contributing to this loss of height is poor posture. When the bones grow weaker, the muscles and bones of the spine bow under the weight of the body, and the individual develops a stooped look referred to by some as "dowager's hump."

ABSORPTION Poor diet or physiological changes can indirectly cause a calcium deficiency; and calcium can be poorly absorbed, too. Ineffective absorption can be caused by smoking, excessive alcohol consumption, magnesium or aluminum-based antacids, some foods, and certain prescriptive drugs. Smoking also increases the risk of osteoporosis because studies show that women who smoke reach menopause several years earlier than nonsmokers, and menopause is a period of increased bone loss.

One factor that can positively affect calcium absorption is exercise. People who do not engage in exercise, especially weight-bearing exercise, a special concern for the bedridden, appear to be less able to replace the calcium they use. Researchers have made the case that it is the lack of weight on the bones that accounts for the negative calcium balance.

Swimming, therefore, does not offer as much benefit as jogging. This phenomenon may account for the fact that the more active people among the elderly population do not have the same degree of bone loss as the less active.

Other positive factors in calcium absorption are vitamin D, a proper gastric acid medium, and a relative balance between calcium and phosphorus. Vitamin D (see page 61) is necessary in the production of a "carrier" protein that takes calcium across the cells of the intestinal walls to the blood. Consequently, a poor vitamin D level results in poor calcium absorption.

Gastric acid, more specifically hydrochloric acid, makes calcium more easily absorbed in the small intestine, which explains why the elderly, who produce less hydrochloric acid, seem to absorb calcium less efficiently. The mineral phosphorus is needed in at least the same amount as calcium because the calcium is absorbed more readily in the presence of phosphorus. On the other hand, if the mineral is consumed in excess, calcium absorption is reduced. On a positive note, vitamin C and magnesium aid in calcium absorption.

WHO IS AT RISK   Perhaps the most common and, at the same time, most serious symptom of a calcium deficiency is bone loss, a problem thought to afflict as many as 15 to 20 million Americans. The group most directly affected are postmenopausal women, and observers believe that the incidence of this deficiency is on the rise. The rate of bone loss in postmenopausal women is considered twice that in men. In general, women have a lower bone mass than men, they consume less calcium-rich food (primary dairy products), and they do less bone-building weight-bearing exercise.

Fifteen to 25 percent of most adult Americans drink little or no milk, our principal dietary source of calcium. Teenage girls consume on the average only 80 percent of the RDA and, in specific cases, tens of thousands of these young women are consuming far less than 80 percent.

Men appear to consume more calcium than women. Some surveys suggest, however, that as many as 20 to 40 percent of American men also take in less than 80 percent. And women between the ages of thirty-five and seventy-four ingest less than two-thirds of the recommended amount.

RECOMMENDED DIETARY ALLOWANCES The RDA for calcium is 800 milligrams, yet many experts recommend that most people get about 1,000 milligrams daily and that all women consume 1,200 milligrams per day. The elderly and women who have reached menopause should consume 1,500 milligrams per day. In the face of this need for calcium, it is unfortunate that the estimated average intake of dietary calcium in this country is not much more than 500 milligrams. Just 12 ounces of cottage cheese or one and a half cups of ice cream represent 500 milligrams of calcium.

It is preferable that calcium needs be met from calcium-rich foods since calcium in this form is more easily absorbed than calcium supplements. For the millions of people unable or unwilling to consume sufficient amounts of calcium-rich foods (studies show that some 70 percent of Blacks and 20 percent of people of European ancestry have trouble ingesting milk), it is recommended that they take a supplement such as calcium carbonate or calcium malate (see Calcium Supplements, page 155) which is known to be well absorbed.

In general, calcium is inefficiently absorbed; perhaps as little as 25 percent of the calcium in the foods adults eat is retained. While rapidly growing children absorb as much as 75 percent of the calcium they consume, the average adult absorbs from 20 to 30 percent, and postmenopausal women as little as 7 percent. What is not absorbed or retained is excreted in the urine or feces, and the rest is lost in perspiration.

ROLE OF EXERCISE It is well documented that long periods of inactivity will cause calcium not to be retained by the bones even though it has been absorbed. If the calcium is not deposited in the bones, it is excreted. Those who suffer from this problem are not only the bedridden but people who lead sedentary lives.

In order for calcium to be properly deposited in bones, the bones have to be stressed through exercise. When the bones are stressed, more calcium is laid down; in other words, the bones grow larger. The exercise must be weight-bearing, however, in order to cause the proper stress on the frame of the body. An example would be an hour of walking; something more strenuous, such as tennis or jogging, would be even better. This is one reason why astronauts, when in a state of weightlessness, lose a measurable amount of calcium from their bones.

Exercise also improves the flow of blood to the bones, thereby increasing the availability of other bone-building nutrients, such as iron. Another benefit of such exercise is that it is thought to produce an electrical discharge within the bones that stimulates bone growth.

Swimming is not an effective form of exercise to prevent bone loss. Swimming places little pressure on the bones because you are suspended in water. It may have excellent cardiovascular benefits and is good for muscle tone, but swimming does not build strong bones.

PROBLEMS OF TOO MUCH CALCIUM Some people take too many calcium supplements. Though an excessive amount of calcium in the blood, hypercalcemia (*hyper* means high, *calc* means calcium, and *emia* means blood), is rare among adults, reasonable amounts of calcium should not be exceeded because too much of it can cause other problems. For example, magnesium directly competes with calcium for absorption. More than 2,000 milligrams of calcium daily could reduce the amount of magnesium absorbed, resulting in a deficiency. Generally, a varied diet guards against this likelihood because magnesium is found in most foods. Another problem associated with excessive levels of calcium is calcium accumulation in soft tissue. Specifically, if you have a predisposition for kidney or gall stones, or suffer from atherosclerosis, which is a hardening of the arteries, excessive calcium supplementation could only worsen these conditions.

Vitamin D, which is stored in the body, increases the absorption of calcium; therefore, if you take excessive amounts of vitamin D, which would be more than 1,000 IU, it will only exacerbate the problem of too much calcium. This would be true whether you are taking an excessive amount of calcium or not. Ten minutes of direct sunlight on your face provides enough vitamin D for the day. (See Vitamin D, page 63).

In animal studies, high intakes of calcium have depressed utilization of other nutrients such as copper, iodine, zinc, and iron. Though there is no evidence that such an inefficient use of these minerals would occur in humans who are taking gross megadoses of calcium, it is certainly possible.

STRATEGIES

FOOD SOURCES   There are a limited number of foods in which calcium is found in significant amounts. The richest source of calcium is dairy products, and this includes low-fat yogurt and hard cheeses. Skim milk is preferred over whole milk since it has fewer calories and more calcium per serving. For the same reasons cottage cheese is preferred over cream cheese. Other good sources are sardines, canned salmon, cauliflower, dark green leafy vegetables, and rhubarb. Poor sources are most fruits, grains, and other vegetables.

The contribution of various foods in our diet to calcium needs are as follows: 75 percent from dairy products; 7 percent from fish, meats, eggs, and vegetables; about 11 percent from the balance of our diet.

As was mentioned before, a calcium deficiency can arise if the ratio of phosphorus to calcium in our diet is too much in favor of phosphorus. Processed foods, especially carbonated beverages, are particularly high in phosphorus. The ideal ratio is 1 to 1 as in dairy products; when the ratio is as high as 20 to 1, as in meat, very little calcium is absorbed. For example, meals high in fat, protein, caffeine, and sodium can contribute to a calcium deficiency, and even a high-fiber diet would cause some problems since fiber is capable of binding to calcium and passing it out in the stool.

DRUG INTERACTIONS Corticosteroids (steroids), which are powerful antiinflammatory drugs, can adversely affect calcium absorption because the long-term use of the drug impairs the activation of vitamin D. They also decrease the absorption of phosphorus, which only exacerbates the calcium loss.

Diphenylmethane Cathartics are laxatives that reduce the time required for the nutrients of food to pass through the wall of the intestines, and thereby they impair calcium absorption.

Ethacrynic Acid and Sodium Ethacrynate, Furosemide, Spironolactone, and Thiazides are all diuretics whose action increases excretion of water and also increases the loss of calcium. The prolonged use of mercurial diuretics (Diamox, Daranide, and Neptazane) could also conceivably lead to a deficiency of calcium.

An anticancer drug called Methotrexate (Folex and Mexate) causes a widespread malabsorption of all nutrients because it damages the intestinal lining. If taken over time it could conceivably cause a calcium deficiency. The same problem of malabsorption is created by the use of mineral oil, a common laxative for many people. Another category of laxatives called Potassium-based Saline Cathartics will also cause problems with calcium absorption.

Long-term use of Isoniazid (INH and Rifamate) and Cycloserine (Seromycin), antitubercular drugs, could conceivably cause a calcium deficiency because they interfere with calcium absorption.

The antibiotics Erythromycin and Tetracycline will impair the absorption of calcium. Ironically, people taking Tetracycline are cautioned not to consume dairy products, which are the best sources for calcium, while taking the drug because the calcium will bind with the drug and prevent it from being absorbed as well.

Antacids containing Magnesium Hydroxide (for example, Milk of Magnesia, Gelusil, and Maalox) can cause an excessive depletion of both phosphate and calcium if used over extended periods.

CALCIUM SUPPLEMENTS It is recommended that you take your calcium supplements in two doses, one taken between meals and the other before you go to bed, because most of the calcium loss from your body occurs while you sleep. Since only 30 percent of the supplement Calcium Carbonate is calcium, it is advised that you take the recommended 1,000 milligrams of calcium in the form of 2,500 milligrams of Calcium Carbonate. If the supplement constipates you, take one that contains magnesium with the calcium.

It is recommended, however, that you don't take calcium as bone meal or dolomite since both could contain lead. Lead consumed in the diet of any animal is stored in the bones. If an animal has been grazing on pastures contaminated by lead from industrial wastes or the environment, their bones could contain some of that lead. On the other hand, dolomite is a mineral that is mined, and it can contain lead impurities. Since the FDA does not monitor the purity of all the bone meal and dolomite sold retail in his country, it is advisable that you take calcium in the form of Calcium Carbonate. Calcium absorption is affected by a substance called oxalic acid, which is found in some foods. If you have reason to believe that calcium deficiency may be a problem, and this would be especially true if you were taking medication that is known to deplete calcium, try to avoid foods such as collard greens, kale, spinach, rhubarb, and chocolate, especially when you are taking calcium supplements.

PHOSPHORUS

DESCRIPTION

Phosphorus is required to keep the acidity of the blood at normal levels, and it is essential to utilization of carbohydrates, fats, and protein for the growth, repair, and reproduction of cells. Coupled with calcium it is necessary for the formation of strong bones and teeth, the transference of nerve impulses, and the contraction of muscles. It is also important to proper kidney functioning, and it is involved with the transference of hereditary traits from parents to offspring. Without phosphorus, niacin (B3) and riboflavin (B2) cannot be digested.

FOOD SOURCES

Excellent sources: meat (especially liver and kidneys), fish, poultry, eggs, cheese, and milk
Good sources: nuts, legumes (beans in a pod), whole grains, dried fruit, and vegetables

HIGH-RISK GROUPS FOR POSSIBLE DEFICIENCY

- people on a severe low-calorie diet
- alcoholics
- people suffering from a wasting disease
- chronic users of antacids (that contain magnesium or aluminum)
- people over the age of 55
- premature infants that are breast-fed
- people with kidney or liver disorders
- people who take megadoses of vitamin D or calcium

RECOMMENDED DOSAGE

GROUP	MG	GROUP	MG
Pregnant women	1,200	Children 7–10	800
Lactating women	1,200	Young women 11–18	1,200
Infants 0.05	240	Adult women 19+	800
0.5–1	360	Young men 11–18	1,200
Children 1–3	800	Adult men 19+	800
4–6	800		

UPPER LIMITS FOR REGULAR DIETARY SUPPLEMENT USE

Children under the age of 4: 1,250 mg
Adults and children 4 or more years of age: 1,500 mg
Pregnant or lactating women: 1,500 mg

TOXIC LEVELS

Have not been established.

BENEFITS

TREATING DEFICIENCY SYMPTOMS
- persistent vomiting
- weakness
- loss of appetite
- pain in the bones
- depression
- muscle tremors
- osteomalacia

UNPROVEN BENEFITS (UNRELATED TO DEFICIENCY SYMPTOMS)

- treatment of arthritic pain
- accelerates growth in children
- treatment of cancer
- treatment of colitis

TOXIC SYMPTOMS

Shortness of breath, irregular heartbeat, seizures, and coma.

DISCOVERY   A German chemist named Hennig Brand was probably the first person to have discovered an element that was not known in any form before his time. He first isolated this nonmetallic element somewhere between 1669 and 1675 by evaporating urine and distilling it. What he obtained was a white, waxy substance that glowed in the dark. Much was made of this discovery because, in addition to glowing in the dark, it broke out into fire when exposed to air. Brand appropriately called this element phosphorus, from two Greek words: *phos,* which means light, and *phoros,* which means carrying.

ROLE   Phosphorus could be considered the most important nutrient in our body, if for no other reason than it plays more roles in the proper functioning of the body than probably any other. It is present in every cell and is involved with almost every metabolic reaction in the body.

Phosphates are important in the maintenance of an acid-base balance in the blood (see Acid-Base Balance, page 149) and in the controlled release of energy resulting from the oxidation of carbohydrates, fats, and protein. Phosphates also make it possible for many nutrients to pass through the cell membrane or to be carried in the blood. Phosphorus is also important in the transmission of nerve impulses.

Because phosphorus is usually found with calcium in the body, the ratio between these two nutrients is critical to their proper functioning. (An ideal calcium-to-phosphorus ratio would be 1 to 1, but realistically 1 to 2 is more than acceptable.) With calcium, phosphorus has an important role in the formation and strengthening of tissues, bones, including the calcification of teeth. In fact, about 80 percent of the phosphorus in the body is stored in the bones and teeth; the remaining 20 percent is found in the blood and tissues.

Some vitamins and enzymes cannot function properly without phosphorus, particularly thiamin (B1), riboflavin (B2), and niacin (B3). Finally, phosphorus is an essential part of the nucleic acids DNA and RDA, which are important to a number of functions including the transference of hereditary traits from parents to offspring.

PROBLEMS OF TOO LITTLE A deficiency of phosphorus is seldom seen because the element is so widely distributed in both plant and animal food. People who have developed a deficiency are those who frequently take antacids, especially antacids that contain magnesium or aluminum hydroxide because the magnesium binds with the phosphorus to form magnesium phosphate, which is eliminated in the stool. The aluminum also blocks the intestinal absorption of phosphorus.

The signs of a phosphorus deficiency are very similar to a calcium deficiency, and in some cases they are identical: loss of appetite, general weakness, muscle tremors, bone pains, and demineralization of the bones. Since these minerals work hand in hand, if you experience a deficiency of one, you will usually have a deficiency of the other.

Chronically low levels of phosphorus can lead to osteomalacia, which is a softening of the bones as a result of losing both calcium and phosphorus. (See Problems of Too Little Calcium, page 150).

WHO IS AT RISK Someone who vomits persistently and consequently is unable to absorb nutrients may be at risk of developing a phosphorus deficiency. People with kidney or liver disorders that produce excessive urinary loss often have had a history of phosphorus deficiencies. Alcoholics also have a variety of nutrient deficiencies, and phosphorus is one of them. Because of its association with calcium, a malabsorption of vitamin D may lead to low phosphorus levels. Finally, people who are on nonphosphate-containing intravenous fluids in the hospital can develop a deficiency.

There are several arguments in favor of breast-feeding infants, two of which are the naturally favorable calcium-to-phosphorus ratio and the low-sodium content of breast milk. (The kidneys of infants have difficulty handling excess sodium.) However, premature infants usually require more phosphorus than is provided in human milk. In fact, because human milk provides only about one-sixth the amount found in cow's milk, some breast-fed premature infants have exhibited a phosphorus deficiency.

TOO MUCH PHOSPHORUS   The ratio of calcium to phosphorus is critical since an increase in one creates a *de facto* deficiency in the other. Phosphorus overload is difficult to achieve through dietary means alone; however, in addition to the sizable consumption of phosphorus-containing carbonated drinks in this country, food additives also contribute to our intake of phosphorus.

Phosphorus is found in most snack or convenience foods, but there is no reason to believe that moderate use of these foods will cause a health problem. Excessive reliance on such foods, however, coupled with a diet that lacks calcium/phosphorus-rich foods, could negatively affect the absorption of calcium and iron.

STRATEGIES

FOOD SOURCES   Phosphorus is found not only in all cells of the body but it is found virtually in all foods. It is chiefly associated with protein-rich foods and cereal products.

Organ meats, such as kidney and liver, are excellent sources, as are fish, poultry, eggs, cheese, and milk. Generally, food products made from grain are good, especially whole-grain foods. Vegetables are adequate sources, but fruits provide only fair amounts of phosphorus.

NOTE   Calcium and phosphorus appear in many of the same foods. They are evenly distributed in some, such as milk, and unevenly in others, such as meat. Among plants they are evenly distributed but not always in the same place on all plants. For example, phosphorus and calcium are found together in relatively the same quantities in the roots, stems, and flowerets of many plants (for example, broccoli), but calcium is more apt to be found in the leaf, whereas phosphorus is in the seeds (or grains) of the plant.

The distribution of phosphorus in the average diet is as follows: 29 percent in meat, fish, and poultry; 34 percent in dairy products; 13 percent in cereal products; 9 percent and 6 percent respectively in vegetables and beans; 5 percent in eggs; and about 4 percent in other foods.

DRUG INTERACTIONS   Antacids that contain Magnesium Hydroxide (Milk of Magnesia, Gelusil, and Maalox) can cause an excessive depletion of both phosphate (phosphorus) and calcium if used over extended periods. Calcium-containing antacids can also decrease the absorption of phosphate.

As much as vitamin D may help the absorption of phosphorus (and calcium), megadoses of vitamin D may create a problem of too much phosphate in the blood. Excessive intake of calcium supplements may also create a deficiency problem for phosphorus.

Diphenylmethane Cathartics, which are laxatives, can cause a general malabsorption problem for many nutrients. While taking these laxatives it is conceivable that they may cause a vitamin D deficiency that could indirectly affect phosphorus. This is more likely if the person has other problems related to a potential deficiency, such as alcoholism. Excessive alcohol consumption may create a deficiency problem because it depletes the body's stores of magnesium, which is needed for phosphorus absorption.

SUPPLEMENTS Phosphorus supplements should be taken only under a doctor's supervision.

POTASSIUM

DESCRIPTION

Potassium is an essential mineral that is found primarily within the cell. With sodium, it helps regulate the distribution of fluids in and out of the cell, and it is critical to the electrolyte balance in the body. It is necessary for stimulation of nerve impulses for muscle contraction (including the heart muscle), and it aids the release of energy from carbohydrates and protein.

FOOD SOURCES

Excellent sources: dried apricots, avocados, flounder, lima beans, black-eyed peas, bananas, oranges, seedless raisins, and dates

Good sources: skim milk, chicken, baked potatoes, pineapples, strawberries, peanut butter, plain yogurt, red meat, clams, and brussels sprouts

HIGH-RISK GROUPS FOR POSSIBLE DEFICIENCY

- people who persistently vomit (for example, bulimics)
- people who suffer from chronic or infectious diarrhea
- people suffering from hyperaldosteronism
- people who use diuretics regularly
- people on long-term fasts
- people suffering from an intestinal obstruction
- people who sweat profusely, such as athletes
- people on severe low-calorie reducing diets (for example, anorexia nervosa)
- heavy users of laxatives
- users of Gentamicin Sulfate, an antibiotic
- users of Sodium Polystyrene Sulfonate (Kayexalate), a drug used for detoxification
- users of Levodopa (Larodopa and Sinemet), a drug to treat Parkinson's disease
- users of Cisplatin (Platinol), an anticancer drug
- users of Digitalis preparations, heart drugs
- users of steroids

RECOMMENDED DOSAGE

GROUP	MG*	GROUP	MG*
Infants 0–0.5	350–925	Children 7–10	1,000–3,000
0.5–1	425–1,275	Young Adults 11–22	1,525–4,575
Children 1–3	550–1,650	Adults 23+	1,875–5,625
4–6	775–2,325		

* These RDAs apply only to potassium. Potassium supplements contain other minerals or elements (such as potassium phosphate), and each of them will have their own RDAs.

TOXIC LEVELS
Have not been established.

BENEFITS
TREATING DEFICIENCY SYMPTOMS
- loss of appetite
- constipation
- muscle weakness
- fatigue
- apathy
- mental confusion
- depression

UNPROVEN BENEFITS (UNRELATED TO DEFICIENCY SYMPTOMS)
- treatment of rickets
- treatment of polio

TOXIC SYMPTOMS
Irregular heartbeat, shortness of breath, and heart failure.

DISCOVERY Sir Humphry Davy, the great English chemist who was the first to discover several minerals, identified potassium in 1807 as a primary element. Any understanding of its nutritional value is of more recent origin. In 1885 experiments established that animal tissues could be maintained in solutions that contained potassium with calcium and sodium in the form of chlorides, which strongly suggested their necessity in sustaining life. Some years later it was determined that the potassium salts found in blood samples were designed for specific, though as yet unknown, functional purposes.

ROLE As a whitish, silvery metal, potassium looks something like sodium and is one of the more abundant elements in the body. It is primarily concentrated within the cell, whereas sodium is primarily outside the cell.

As an integral part of the cell, potassium is essential to growth. In addition to constituting 5 percent of the total mineral content of the body, it is thought that for every pound of weight added, a little more than 1,000 milligrams is required. Within the cell, potassium acts as a cofactor in the synthesis of protein. It is important in the conversion of glucose to glycogen, which permits the glucose to be stored in the liver for potential energy uses. The electrical potential of all cell membranes and the conduction of nerve impulses rely on potassium (and sodium).

A dramatic example of the importance of this mineral (and magnesium) is the fact that the proper functioning of heart tissue requires potassium. Too little or too much potassium can cause the heart to stop. For this reason potassium supplements are prescribed for many people whose hearts do not pump enough blood, a condition known as heart failure.

PROBLEMS OF TOO LITTLE   It is not clear as to how little potassium adults need; however, it is estimated to be about 2 grams per day. (The RDA minimum is precisely 1,875 milligrams.) What the average diet provides is thought to be between 2,000 to 6,000 milligrams, which basically ensures most people an adequate supply of the mineral. If a deficiency develops, it is usually characterized by poor intestinal muscle tone, especially abdominal bloating, and by heart abnormalities and a weakness of respiratory muscles. A condition that poses a threat of too little potassium is called *hyperaldosteronism*. Small tumors present in the adrenal gland can produce this disorder, which is an overproduction of the hormone aldosterone. An excessive amount of this most powerful of the salt-retaining hormones can lead to a depletion of potassium (and too much sodium). A potassium deficiency should be treated by a physician, and potassium supplements should not be taken without a doctor's supervision.

WHO IS AT RISK   A pure dietary deficiency of potassium is unlikely in a healthy person since the mineral is found widely in foods. A deficiency is more likely to occur during certain illnesses or under conditions of ill health, such as chronic diarrhea, persistent vomiting, or if certain medications are prescribed that can increase potassium excretion, such as diuretics.

Infants may develop a deficiency if they suffer from diarrhea because the food passes through their intestine so quickly that its nutrients cannot be absorbed. Someone who suffers from bulimia, an eating disorder that involves induced vomiting after eating enormous amounts of food, is at risk of a potential potassium deficiency.

TOO MUCH   Excess potassium is excreted in the urine by the action of the kidneys. Much in the same way in which the kidneys regulate the sodium content of the body, kidneys can regulate fairly large differences of potassium intake by reabsorbing it into the body or excreting in the urine. This system permits the body to maintain a stable and important concentration of potassium in the cell. This does not mean, however, that potassium supplements can be taken willy-nilly. Excessive concentrations in the bloodstream can be dangerous because they can cause an abnormal heartbeat or heart failure.

Excess potassium in the blood, called *hyperkalemia,* may produce symptoms such as muscle weakness, mental confusion, cold and pale skin, and seizures. Cases of hyperkalemia are rare, but they can occur if too much potassium is taken in the form of supplements or if someone is suffering from kidney failure.

The elderly have a special problem with excessively high blood levels of potassium because many of them have impaired kidney function which can prevent their kidneys from excreting sufficient amounts of the mineral.

STRATEGIES

FOOD SOURCES Most foods contain some potassium, with the exception of sugar and fats. The foods richest in potassium are citrus fruits (for example, oranges and pineapples), apricots, bananas, cantaloupe, dates, figs, peaches, prunes, raisins, and tomatoes. Beef, veal, pork, beef liver, the white meat of chicken, and canned pink salmon are good sources. Among vegetables and legumes (peas in a pod), good sources are lima beans, black-eyed peas, broccoli, brussels sprouts, carrots, green peas, and potatoes. On the other hand, foods such as cheese, eggs, and cereals are only moderate sources of potassium.

FOOD PREPARATION Because of the generous abundance of potassium in our diet, its destruction in food preparation is not as critical as is the case of vitamin destruction. It should be pointed out, however, that methods of food preservation and cooking tend to deplete some foods of potassium. For example, since potassium is very soluble, considerable amounts of potassium can be leached if boiled for long periods in large amounts of water.

DRUG INTERACTIONS Anthraquinone Cathartics and Diphenylmethane Cathartics, which are laxatives, cause potassium to pass into the digestive tract where it is excreted. If mineral oils are used regularly as a laxative, they can create a similar malabsorption of potassium.

Diuretics such as Ethacrynic Acid and Sodium Ethacrynate, Furosemide, Thiazides, and Spironolactone, impair the body's ability to absorb potassium and increase its rate of excretion. Long-term use of Mercurial Diuretics can also result in a potassium depletion.

Corticosteroids (steroids) increase the rate of excretion of potassium, and the antibiotic Gentamicin Sulfate could negatively affect the kidneys and cause a loss of potassium (and magnesium).

Sodium Polystyrene Sulfonate (Kayexalate), a drug used for detoxification, can directly cause a potassium deficiency, and a drug for treating Parkinson's disease, Levodopa (Larodopa and Sinemet) also increases the excretion of potassium.

Cisplatin (Platinol), an anticancer drug, can cause a potassium deficiency.

Digitalis preparations, drugs that increase the force at which the heart pumps, also negatively affect potassium levels.

Some other drugs, such as penicillin, may mildly increase potassium excretion or create some minor problem of potassium absorption, but not to any extent that is noteworthy.

MAGNESIUM

DESCRIPTION
Magnesium is involved in many metabolic reactions in the body. It activates enzymes necessary for metabolism of carbohydrates and amino acids. It also helps to regulate the acid-alkaline balance in the body, and it promotes the absorption and metabolism of other minerals such as calcium, phosphorus, sodium, and potassium. Bone growth depends on magnesium, and it is essential to proper functioning of nerves and muscles.

FOOD SOURCES
Excellent sources: dry mustard, cashew nuts, cow peas, peanut butter, curry powder, and instant coffee
Good sources: spinach, whole-grain breads, graham crackers, snap beans, cheddar cheese, and bananas

HIGH-RISK GROUPS FOR POSSIBLE DEFICIENCY
- people on a severe low-calorie diet
- people suffering from a wasting disease
- alcoholics
- people recovering from post-surgery stress or severe burns
- people suffering from hyperthyroidism and diseases of the parathyroid
- people suffering from severe infections
- people suffering from chronic gastrointestinal disorders
- people with diabetes
- people undergoing renal (kidney) therapy
- people taking diuretics
- people taking several antitubercular drugs
- people taking the antibiotics Gentamicin Sulfate (Garamycin), Sulfisoxazole, and Sulfamethoxazole
- people taking digitalis preparations such as Crystodigin, and Lanoxicaps, and Lanoxin, drugs to treat a heart condition
- people taking the anticancer drug Cisplatin (Platinol)

RECOMMENDED DOSAGE

GROUP	MG	GROUP	MG
Pregnant women	450	Children 7–10	250
Lactating women	450	Young women 11–22	300
Infants 0–0.5	50	Adult women 23+	300
0.5–1	70	Young men 11–14	350
Children 1–3	150	15–18	400
4–6	200	Adult men 19+	350

UPPER LIMITS OF REGULAR DIETARY SUPPLEMENT USE

Children under 4 years of age: 300 mg
Adults and children over 4 years of age: 600 mg
Pregnant or lactating women: 800 mg

TOXIC LEVELS

Have not been established.

BENEFITS

TREATING DEFICIENCY SYMPTOMS

- poor bone growth
- muscle spasms
- nausea
- apathy
- anorexia
- constipation
- excessive stomach acid (in small doses)
- nervousness and irritability

OTHER POSSIBLE BENEFITS
- in the treatment of heart disease

UNPROVEN BENEFITS (UNRELATED TO DEFICIENCY SYMPTOMS)

- cures kidney stones
- cures alcoholism
- treats multiple sclerosis
- treats obesity and body odor
- reduces cholesterol levels

TOXIC SYMPTOMS

Loss of reflexes, drowsiness, depression, and coma.

DISCOVERY   For centuries magnesium had been believed to be a healing substance. The Romans claimed that *magnesia alba,* which means white magnesium, cured a wide variety of ailments. It probably was used as an anticonvulsant and an anesthetic.

Sir Humphry Davy, the great English chemist, is credited with first isolating the mineral in 1808, and a German chemist, Robert Wilhelm Bunsen (of Bunsen burner fame), was the first to produce magnesium in large quantities in the middle of the nineteenth century. The presence of magnesium was discovered in the human body about 1850, and ten years later it was determined that it was essential to plant life. But it was not until 1926 that magnesium was proved to be an essential nutrient in the human body. The basis for this assumption grew out of the work of a French chemist, Jean Leroy, who established the reasons magnesium was essential for mice. A few years later American chemists determined the existence of magnesium deficiencies in rats and dogs, including a deficiency condition they called magnesium tetany. (Tetany is a condition in which muscles intermittently relax and contract because of low blood levels of calcium—see Calcium, page 150).

Only since 1950 have we come to learn the various roles magnesium plays in human nutrition. This seeming delay in determining the human need for magnesium was due to the difficulty in studying the effects of a magnesium deficiency since methods for measuring magnesium in body fluids were not very sophisticated, and the kidneys had the ability to reabsorb magnesium whenever needed. Once techniques could be developed to measure magnesium levels in the body, however, it was proved that magnesium existed in probably all cell tissue and was an essential element to their growth.

ROLE Magnesium is associated with hundreds of metabolic reactions in the cell. Its principal role is in the formation of bone structure since more than half of the body's stores of magnesium are found in bone. By activating numerous enzymes magnesium is also involved in virtually all the reactions involving the expenditure or release of energy, especially for muscle contraction, and nerve impulses. The metabolism of carbohydrates, fats, protein, and nucleic acids all depend on magnesium. It is required for the activation of an enzyme that is important in the metabolism of calcium and phosphorus.

Magnesium is necessary for protein synthesis and the synthesis and degradation of DNA. Many other functions in the body are affected by its extensive interrelationships with calcium, phosphorus, potassium, sodium, parathyroid hormone, and vitamin D. Its relationship with calcium is one of interdependence. Calcium appears to affect the kidney's ability to reabsorb magnesium, while magnesium helps to liberate needed calcium from the bones for use in the cells. Magnesium excretion also decreases as calcium is reduced.

PROBLEMS OF TOO LITTLE Magnesium requirements will vary depending on the size and composition of the individual's diet. A great amount of calcium in the diet is known to compete with the absorption of magnesium; therefore, excess consumption of calcium will reduce the absorption of magnesium. Increased amounts of protein, phosphorus, and vitamin D can also increase magnesium requirements.

One recognizable sign of a serious deficiency is a condition called low magnesium tetany, which begins with muscle tremors and progresses until convulsions occur. Another symptom is the calcification or hardening of soft tissue. This deficiency symptom probably reflects an increase in calcium due to the reduced magnesium available to compete with it for absorption.

Some people flush, or their skin grows reddish, during a magnesium deficiency. These symptoms may be explained by the fact that inadequate amounts of magnesium result in vasodilation, an increase in the size of blood vessels. Consequently, when more blood flows through the expanded blood vessels, those near the surface of the skin cause it to appear reddish.

In the past it has been difficult to measure magnesium levels in body fluids with any accuracy, but with new methods available it is thought that magnesium depletions are more common than previously understood.

WHO IS AT RISK Deficiencies are not common, but they occur among people suffering from specific illnesses, especially kidney disorders, or among those recovering from intestinal surgery. People on certain drugs are also exposed to a possible deficiency, especially those taking diuretics.

It is believed that magnesium intakes are poor for many people, especially those on diets that rely on potatoes, starches, and fatty meats. Adolescent females appear to lose more magnesium than they take in, and the intake for many is thought to be only two-thirds of the RDA. One study indicated that 13 to 35 percent of preteen females consume less than 67 percent of the RDA.

A government survey in 1977 showed that the daily intake of adult women was slightly more than 200 milligrams (RDA is 300 milligrams), and for men it was close to 300 milligrams (RDA is 350 milligrams). Magnesium requirements are higher for women during pregnancy and lactation, too. All this is not necessarily alarming because the body wisely alerts the kidneys to reabsorb almost all magnesium when magnesium intake is low. This conserving function reduces the likelihood that a drop in dietary magnesium will easily affect blood levels. Over an extended period, however, a diet that is poor in magnesium can be the cause of some symptoms, especially in people who experience an illness or condition that causes additional magnesium loss.

NOTE About 30 to 40 percent of the magnesium we ingest is absorbed, unless we have a condition that impairs normal absorption. Newborn infants fare pretty well because, whether breast-fed or bottle-fed, they will absorb as much as 85 percent of the magnesium available in their milk.

Deficiency symptoms are seen in people suffering from persistent vomiting, starvation (anorexia), or from chronic diarrhea. Diarrhea poses a problem because the rapid passage of food through the gastrointestinal tract reduces the time for proper absorption. On occasion deficiencies have occurred with people who have been fed intravenously. (It is called total parenteral feeding.) The cause of the deficiency lies not in the feeding procedure but in the solution that is fed, which apparently did not meet the magnesium needs.

TOO MUCH MAGNESIUM Toxicity can occur in people who suffer from kidney failure because the kidneys are responsible for regulating normal magnesium balance. Toxicity is also seen in people who have received excessive amounts of magnesium salts in clinical situations, such as those being treated for convulsions.

STRATEGIES

FOOD SOURCES It is unlikely that we will ever run out of magnesium as a dietary nutrient because it is estimated that each cubic mile of sea water contains 6 million tons of magnesium.

Its distribution in foods is not as broad, but a normal diet easily provides adequate amounts. Magnesium appears in many foods that are relatively poor in calories; for example, some of the best sources are instant cocoa, coffee, and tea (in dry powder form), dry powdered mustard, baking chocolate, and curry powder. When it comes to more nutritious foods, the best choices, aside from peanut butter, nuts (such as cashews), and cowpeas, are vegetables. Foods such as legumes, seafood, cereal, and dairy products are also good selections for magnesium content.

In years past the "hard" water we drank was an abundant supply of magnesium. Two quarts of hard water might have provided as much as 240 milligrams of magnesium. But today much of our drinking water has been appropriately treated or softened, which means much of the magnesium has been removed, along with such toxic elements as lead, cadmium, pesticides, herbicides, and industrial wastes that may have seeped in.

The distribution of magnesium in the average diet is as follows: 22 percent comes from our vegetables and fruit; cereal products provide 21 percent; meat, poultry, fish, and eggs, 20 percent; dairy products, 17 percent; nonalcoholic beverages, 12 percent, and legumes, about 5 percent; the balance, 3 percent, comes from desserts, chocolate, and other foods.

FOOD PREPARATION   The processing of foods can produce considerable loss of magnesium; for example, white polished rice is very poor, and white flour yields about only one-fifth the magnesium content found in whole-grain cereals. There is practically no magnesium in sugar, alcohol, fats, and oils. The practice of boiling vegetables not only destroys several water-soluble vitamins but it causes a loss of magnesium as well. If vegetables are boiled, the best advice is to save and use the water in the preparation of other foods because it retains many of the vitamins and all of the "lost" magnesium.

DRUG INTERACTIONS   A magnesium deficiency resulting from any one of the drugs listed below is not probable. If someone is borderline deficient, however, due to some other condition or is taking a diuretic, the risk of a deficiency with these drugs is increased.

Ethacrynic Acid and Sodium Ethacrynate, Furosemide (Lasix and SK-Furosemide), and Thiazides are all diuretics that can impair magnesium absorption. This is also true of the Mercurial Diuretics (Diamox, Daranide, and Neptazane).

The anticancer drug called Cisplatin (Platinol) increases magnesium (including potassium and zinc) excretion. Though magnesium deficiencies are rare, the negative effect of this powerful drug on magnesium makes a deficiency a possibility.

Digitalis Preparations—Digitalis Glycoside (Crystodigin) and Digoxin (Lanoxicaps) and (Lanoxin)—to treat a heart condition may increase the risk of a magnesium deficiency.

The antibiotics Gentamicin Sulfate (Garamycin), Sulfisoxazole, and Sulfamethoxazole impair the absorption of magnesium. Isoniazid (INH and Rifamate), Cycloserine (Seromycin), and Para-Aminosalicylic Acid, used for the treatment of tuberculosis, decrease the absorption of several vitamins and minerals, one of which is magnesium.

SODIUM

DESCRIPTION
About half of the total body sodium, an essential mineral, is found inside the fluid of cells, and the balance outside the cell is found primarily in blood vessels, arteries, veins, capillaries, and intestinal fluids. Some is also found in the skeleton. Along with potassium, sodium helps balance the acid-alkaline content of blood and regulate the distribution of body fluids. It is involved with muscle contraction and expansion, and with nerve stimulation. With chlorine it is important to the health of the blood and lymph, helps purge carbon dioxide from the body, and aids in digestion. As sodium chloride, it is necessary to hydrochloride production in the gastric juice.

FOOD SOURCES
Excellent sources: anchovies, sardines, cooked ham, sausage, bacon, beans, dill pickles, cheddar and Parmesan cheeses
Good sources: tomato juice, clams, canned peas, green olives, canned beets, canned corn, cooked scallops, and buttermilk

HIGH-RISK GROUPS FOR POSSIBLE DEFICIENCY
- people with a kidney disorder
- people who suffer from chronic diarrhea
- people suffering from adrenal insufficiency
- heavy users of diuretics
- people who sweat profusely

RECOMMENDED DOSAGE
The dietary requirement for sodium has not been determined but the usual intake far exceeds what is needed.

TOXIC LEVELS
Have not been established.

BENEFITS

TREATING DEFICIENCY SYMPTOMS

The possibility of a naturally occurring sodium deficiency is rare.

MODERATE DEFICIENCY

- loss of appetite
- weight loss

- irritability
- general weakness

GROSS DEFICIENCY

- persistent vomiting

- mental confusion

TOXIC SYMPTOMS

Heart failure and coma.

DISCOVERY   Sodium and common salt are not the same, but the terms are often used interchangeably. Sodium is only the basic element, whereas common salt is a compound of sodium (40 percent) and chloride (60 percent).

The value of sodium in the form of salt has a long history. It was prized in the ancient world as a mineral that could both flavor and preserve foods, such as meat and fish. As a valued item of commerce, Roman soldiers were paid their wages in the form of salt or were given money for the purchase of salt. Marco Polo noted in China that cakes of salt impressed with the sign of the khan were used as payment for gold.

Despite the fact that the importance of salt was known for centuries, especially as a seasoning and preservative, the value of sodium (and therefore of common salt) as essential to the human diet was scientifically established only in 1937.

ROLE   Water and therefore sodium is found in three compartments in the body: within the cell, which is called intracellular fluid; outside the cell, which is called extracellular; and as a part of extracellular fluid, the water in the blood is called intravascular.

In addition to sodium being found in all the fluids inside and outside the cells and in the circulating fluids of the body, other minerals, especially potassium, are also in all these fluids. The greater concentration of sodium is in extracellular fluid, however, and potassium has its greatest concentration in the intracellular fluid. The critical balance between these two elements determines the proper water balance in the body.

Whenever sodium and potassium get out of balance, for whatever reason, fluid-bearing sodium moves in, or out, of the cell to correct the problem. This tension of balanced pressures between the fluids inside the cell with fluids outside the cell is called *osmotic pressure*. The word is formed from the Greek *osmos,* which means impulse. Osmotic pressure is what occurs when two solutions are separated by a semipermeable membrane (the wall of the cell) that resists the impulse for the two solutions to pass through and mix.

Sodium, as the predominant positively charged ion in the fluids outside the cell, is responsible for establishing enough pressure to keep the water from leaving the blood and entering the cell. This is one example of osmotic pressure. (The other is the balance between the sodium and potassium of the extracellular and intracellular fluids.)

Sodium is necessary for the transmission of the nerve impulses, which cause the muscles to contract and relax; for the heart, which requires sodium as does the acid-alkaline content of blood; and for the metabolism of proteins and carbohydrates.

ELECTROLYTES Salt is a general term for a compound that contains a positive and negative charge, and this charge takes the form of a particle called an ion. Common salt is a compound made up of two elements that are charged differently: sodium (+) and chloride (−). The salts in the body (for example, sodium chloride and potassium chloride) are called electrolytes, and it is these electrolytes in the fluids of the body that conduct an electric current, much like a battery.

A law of electricity (electrical neutrality) states that the sum of positive ions or charges, called cations, in an electrolyte solution must equal the sum of the negative ions or charges, called anions. Since our body contains compounds that have different charges (for example, sodium and potassium have a positive charge (+), while chlorine has a negative charge (−), the fluids of our body must be balanced between the sum of all the positive and negative charges of all the elements. (See Acid-Base Balance, page 149.)

PROBLEMS OF TOO LITTLE OR TOO MUCH If the amount of sodium is too great within the cell, water will enter it and cause the tissue to swell, creating a condition called *edema*. To keep it balanced the cell must constantly pump out any extra sodium that might tip this delicate balance of water.

SODIUM DEFICIENCY The possibility of a sodium deficiency is quite rare among human beings; however, animal studies have been conducted to learn what kinds of symptoms a lack of sodium might produce. A biochemist at the University of Wisconsin studied the need for salt in animals by giving one half of a dairy herd regular feed and the other half unsalted feed. At first the salt-deprived cows began to lick the soil because of a craving for salt. Eventually, they lost their appetite and weight, gave less milk, and produced weak calves, some of whom did not survive. When sodium was reintroduced to their diet, the cows returned to good health almost immediately.

Humans who have experienced a sodium deficiency because of an illness or kidney disorder exhibit some of the same symptoms as those of test animals, including loss of appetite and weight, irritability, muscle cramps, general weakness, and a loss of thirst. During a severe deficiency, the symptoms are worse and include persistent vomiting, mental confusion, heart failure, and coma.

WHO IS AT RISK   A chronic sodium deficiency is rare because sodium is so readily available in our diet. It is quite rare that someone would eat a diet so deficient in salt that it could produce deficiency symptoms. Nevertheless, cases of acute sodium depletion are reported, usually among people with severe diarrhea, kidney disease, or those who develop a condition called Addison's disease or adrenal insufficiency.

People who sweat profusely can lose a great deal of salt. Athletes are known to lose as much as fifteen pounds during the course of a game—which is principally water and, of course, sodium chloride. Another example are laborers in the tropics who, it is reported, have lost as much as ten or more quarts of water through perspiration, amounting to a critical loss of ten grams of salt. The kidneys can adjust to these temporary loses, but if sodium intakes are not increased, symptoms of a sodium deficiency soon develop.

TOO MUCH   Small tumors in the adrenal gland can produce a disorder called hyperaldosteronism, an overproduction of the hormone aldosterone. This hormone is the most powerful of the salt-retaining hormones, and an excess can lead to too much sodium, hypertension, and a depletion of potassium.

Sodium toxicity, or salt poisoning, is a rare but very dangerous condition. Among other things, it will damage the kidneys, which can be life-threatening. The relationship of salt to high blood pressure is still not fully understood, but it is believed that sodium restriction apparently helps those already affected by hypertension (which is another word for high blood pressure). This does not mean that salt causes hypertension or that a low-sodium diet will prevent someone from developing the disease. Animal studies have proven a cause-and-effect relationship between salt and hypertension, but there is no conclusive evidence that such a sodium-blood pressure link exists in humans.

A moderate sodium intake is prudent practice, but there is no evidence that indicates the need for healthy people to restrict themselves to 300 milligrams of sodium per day, as some people have suggested.

STRATEGIES

FOOD SOURCES Sodium appears in our diet in three different ways: as a natural ingredient of food; as an additive for flavoring or preserving; added in food preparation in the home.

Many people ignore the fact that sodium is found naturally in nearly all foods. About 25 percent of our average sodium intake comes to us in this fashion. Some well-known examples are anchovies, cooked ham, bacon, and dill pickles. Some other less well-known foods are cheddar and Parmesan cheeses, scallops, clams, canned peas, beets, corn, green olives, eggs, and buttermilk.

Fresh fruits and vegetables are low in sodium, but if these foods are processed, it is very likely that they will contain much more sodium than in their natural state. Commercially prepared cereals and breads contain only moderate amounts of sodium, but soft drinks can be a significant source of sodium.

The approximate distribution of sodium in the average diet is as follows: 29 percent is found in grain and cereal products; 30 percent comes from salt that is added; 14 percent is contributed by meat, poultry, and fish; 11 percent comes from dairy products; vegetables, 8 percent; 6 percent from oils, fats, and shortening; 2 percent comes from fruit and potatoes.

FOOD PREPARATION The principal means of controlling excess salt in your diet is by reducing the amount of salt added during food preparation. It is estimated that the average daily diet contains about 5,000 milligrams of sodium, or 12 grams of common salt. At this rate, the average adult consumes in the course of a year more than nine pounds of salt.

As additives to preserve, flavor, and enhance the color of foods, sodium enters our diet in many different ways: baking powder and baking soda; monosodium glutamate (MSG); sodium alginate (for smooth texture in ice cream); sodium benzoate (as a preservative); brine (in freezing, pickling, and canning); disodium phosphate (in quick-cooking cereals); sodium sulfite (to bleach some fruits or as a preservative in others); sodium hydroxide (to soften skins of foods such as olives, fruits, and vegetables); sodium propionate (to retard mold growth in pasteurized cheeses and pastries).

In addition, some of the nonfoods we consume in our diet contain significant amounts of sodium, such as many antacids.

CHLORIDE

DESCRIPTION

As an essential mineral, chlorine appears in the body as a salt in compound form with sodium (sodium chloride) and potassium (potassium chloride). Chloride is an important anion (a negative-charged ion) in the chemistry of the body. It helps to regulate the correct balance of acid and alkali in the blood, is an essential component of hydrochloric acid necessary for proper digestion, is involved in activating nerve impulses, and permits the blood to carry more carbon dioxide to the lungs.

FOOD SOURCES

The primary source of dietary chlorine is in the compound sodium chloride or common table salt. Foods that contain sodium chloride provide almost exclusively all the chlorine we need. Some water supplies provide as much as 300 milligrams per quart, but usually our drinking water accounts for about 20 milligrams per quart.

HIGH-RISK GROUPS FOR POSSIBLE DEFICIENCY

The same people at risk of a sodium deficiency or who experience a deficiency suffer from a chlorine deficiency.

RECOMMENDED DOSAGE

The RDAs for sodium, in the form of sodium chloride, supply adequate amounts of chlorine.

TOXIC LEVELS

Have not been established.

BENEFITS

TREATING DEFICIENCY SYMPTOMS

The symptoms of a chloride deficiency, which are essentially the same as for a sodium deficiency, include water loss if there is an equal loss of both minerals.

TOXIC SYMPTOMS

There is no known toxic syndrome for chloride, but chlorine gas is so poisonous that it has been used in chemical warfare.

ROLE   Because it is a negative ion, referred to as an *anion,* chlorine is essential to the regulation of the major positive ions (sodium and potassium) to achieve an electrical balance or electrical neutrality in the cells. Along with other acid-forming elements, phosphorus and sulfur, it helps in the acid-base balance in the body fluids. As carbon dioxide is taken up by the blood and released in the lungs, chloride crosses the membrane of the red blood cell to counteract any change in the acid-base balance that might have occurred. This movement of chloride in and out of red blood cells is called *chloride transfer.*

Chloride helps form hydrochloride acid, a principal component of gastric juice that is essential to proper digestion, especially for the metabolism of proteins.

PROBLEMS OF TOO LITTLE   A chloride deficiency might occur only in the presence of a sodium deficiency since our supply of chlorine is almost exclusively through the compound sodium chloride. Chloride is lost chiefly through excretion in the urine, but it is also lost through perspiration and in gastrointestinal secretions.

If health considerations due to heart or kidney disease demand that sodium intake be restricted, chlorine can be consumed in the form of another salt—potassium chloride—but only with a doctor's supervision. Too much potassium can be very dangerous.

WHO IS AT RISK   Because of the compound relationship between sodium and chlorine (sodium chloride), a deficiency of one affects the other; for example, people who experience a sodium deficiency because of severe diarrhea, kidney disease, or a condition called adrenal insufficiency may also experience a chloride deficiency. (Adrenal insufficiency, which is a disorder that causes the adrenal glands to underproduce the hormone aldosterone, can cause a sodium deficiency because the hormone is responsible for retaining salt in the body.)

It is believed that repeated vomiting will not only cause a loss of sodium but the chloride losses may be worse and should be replaced.

STRATEGIES

FOOD SOURCES   Most of the same foods that supply sodium also provide chloride in the form of the compound sodium chloride. (See Sodium, page 173.)

SULFUR

DESCRIPTION

Sulfur is found in every cell and probably makes up about .25 percent of the total body weight. It is part of various organic compounds such as the three vitamins thiamin, pantothenic acid, and biotin. It is also a constituent component of insulin, an anticoagulant called heparin, and it is found in three amino acids: cystine, methionine, and taurine.

The main function of sulfur is in the clotting of blood, in the development of bone, muscle metabolism, and possibly as a growth factor. Some compounds containing sulfur act as a detoxifying substance whereby they combine with the toxic substance to form a harmless compound and are then excreted.

The highest concentrations of sulfur are found in the hair, skin, and nails. (If you have ever smelled burning or burnt hair, the strong odor given off is sulfur dioxide.

Dietary sulfur appears in foods such as beef, dried beans and peas, peanut butter, and wheat germ.

WATER

DESCRIPTION
Water is the most abundant and most important nutrient found in the body. It makes up about 60 percent of the total body weight of an average adult male and 50 percent of an average adult female. (With advancing age the total drops to about 45 percent.) Water is responsible for and involved in nearly every body process including digestion, absorption, circulation, and excretion. It provides transportation throughout the body for many nutrients, ions, and hormones, and it is necessary for many growth functions in the body. It regulates normal body temperature and is essential for carrying waste material out of the body. It also contains and lubricates the joints of the body.

FOOD SOURCES
Excellent sources: watermelon, cucumber, lettuce, raw tomato, celery, milk, and oranges
Good sources: raw oysters, apples, bananas, raw eggs, cooked spaghetti, cooked hamburger, and cheddar cheese

HIGH-RISK GROUPS FOR POSSIBLE DEFICIENCY
- people who suffer from chronic diarrhea
- athletes and people who do heavy exercise in hot weather (especially marathon runners and wrestlers)
- people who suffer from poor kidney function

RECOMMENDED DOSAGE
There are different ways to express our need for water. Under conditions of moderate temperature and exercise, however, an acceptable means of measure is as follows:
Generally, adults should drink 2 quarts of water (or liquids containing water) daily to replace normal losses.

BENEFITS
TREATING DEFICIENCY SYMPTOMS
MILD DEFICIENCY
(a water loss up to 5 percent of total body weight):
- thirst
- vague discomfort or sense of oppression

- loss of appetite
- fatigue or general weariness
- apathy
- flushed skin

GROSS DEFICIENCY
(a water loss more than 5 percent of total body weight):
- tingling in the arms, hands, and feet
- stumbling
- headaches
- increased body temperature, pulse, and respiratory rate
- indistinct speech and mental confusion
- swollen tongue
- delirium
- inability to swallow

TOXIC SYMPTOMS
Water loss of more than 15 percent of total body weight.
Shriveled skin, dim vision, sunken eyes, painful urination, cracked skin and coma. A water loss of more than 20 percent of total body weight will almost certainly be fatal.

ROLE   Without water, human life could not be sustained because water is involved in every chemical reaction that takes place in every cell of the body. The roles of water range from being a solvent for the transportation of nutrients and oxygen to a regulator of body temperature and a cushion for body joints.

Transporter: Water in the body provides the principal form of transportation for most nutrients and many hormones. The nutrients are dissolved in the water of the blood and carried by the bloodstream. As a solvent, water also carries away the waste products of metabolism from the cells to the lungs, skin, or kidneys to be excreted. It also provides transportation for oxygen throughout the entire system. Even the water in the space between the cells, and within the cell itself, carries nutrients and collects waste products.

Catalyst: In the stomach and small intestine, water is required for successful digestion of food. It is also needed in a process by which some complex substances are broken down into two or more simpler components. One example of this process, called hydrolysis, is the action of water on sucrose (one form of sugar) to form glucose and fructose (two other sugars).

Growth Factor: All tissues contain water, which is essential for growth. Water also makes up a significant part of a number of other nutrients. Two-thirds of glycogen (the form in which carbohydrate is stored in the liver) is water; one-fifth of fat tissue is water; and muscle is almost three-fourths water.

Heat Regulator: As a conductor of heat, water can carry heat away from specific areas of the body or carry it to the surface and lose it by the evaporation from the skin. Through evaporation, which is the principal way the body cools itself, the body loses as much as 25 percent of its heat.

Mineral Provider: The source of the drinking water will determine what other elements and how much of them the water contains. Water can be the source of trace elements such as iron, copper, zinc, and fluorine, and macro-elements such as magnesium and calcium.

Cushion or Lubricant: Water acts as a necessary lubricant in pressure areas and joints such as the knee, and it also prevents friction between the bones and ligaments.

WATER LOSS A varied amount of water is used and expelled by the body each day. To maintain a proper balance the input must pretty much match the output. The average turnover in a healthy adult under normal conditions ranges between 2.1 and 3.2 quarts per day. Water is lost or eliminated through the urine and the feces, the skin, and the lungs.

The greatest amount of water in our body is found in our bloodstream. Blood, which is 80 percent water, circulates throughout the body and picks up waste products of metabolism. Most of these waste products are excreted in the urine, which itself is about 97 percent water. The kidneys also use water to maintain normal blood volumes. What is not used is excreted. During normal water intakes, the urine volume should range between one and two quarts. Of course, if intake is increased, so is the volume of urine.

Water is also lost through the skin. Within normal ranges you may lose water at a rate of about 12 to 24 ounces a day. In conditions of high heat and low humidity, or during a fever, water losses will rise. Workers in the tropics have been known to perspire so much that they lost more than ten quarts of water.

Water is also lost through the lungs, along with carbon dioxide. The amount released in this manner is not much more than one cup per day. If respiration rates increase due to exercise or high altitudes, more water is lost. If the air is unusually dry and hot, the total amount of water lost through the lungs and skin may be as high as urinary losses.

A lot of water passes through the gastrointestinal tract in the form of digestive juices. The water used in the digestive process is reabsorbed as it passes through the gastrointestinal tract so that as little as 7 ounces per day may be lost in the feces. The kidneys of a healthy adult filter about 50 gallons of water a day. Most of this is recycled water that is reabsorbed for continued use.

Diarrhea increases the loss of water and other nutrients, and persistent vomiting will result in a high loss of water. If either condition persists, it can cause dehydration, which is a severe problem if the fluid and sodium levels are not restored.

Because water losses vary depending on body weight, activity, and environmental conditions, it is advised that your intake should be about 2 quarts to compensate for normal water losses in the urine, feces, skin, and lungs. Even under conditions of a low solute load (the amount of waste products that needs to be excreted by the kidneys), minimal physical activity, and an absence of sweating, the total water from food and drink should be at least 1.5 quarts per day.

NOTE Small infants lose a higher percentage of water by evaporation from the skin than adults; therefore, extra water should be provided for infants when the temperature is high.

DEHYDRATION A natural exchange of body water occurs continually during the course of each day. Approximately 6 percent of the total volume of water in an adult body is replaced each day, and as much as 15 percent of the total volume in an infant's body is replaced. These exchanges are not the same as net losses, which, of course, are problems if sustained for any period.

Long-term losses of water are always a matter of concern. In fact, a healthy adult can probably live only a few days without water. (The longest anyone has lived without water is thought to be seventeen days.) Whenever water losses occur, the body performs a number of functions to conserve the remaining water, one of which is to alert the brain that intakes should be increased. (The brain's message is to create a desire or thirst for more water.) When the water intake is appropriate, there is no outstanding net loss over any period. If there were a loss, the symptoms would persist and possibly grow worse.

Symptoms: After only a 2 percent loss the body experiences a strong thirst, possibly loss of appetite, and constipation. By the time the net loss reaches 4 percent, the symptoms are flushed skin, impatience, weariness, sleepiness, apathy, and nausea. If the loss were to continue, the symptoms would grow more severe. When a water loss reaches a level of 10 percent of the total body weight, the body begins to experience a general incapacity, including the Romberg sign—an inability to balance with the eyes closed. A loss of 20 percent would be fatal in only a very short period.

NOTE A lack of water may affect work performance more than a lack of food. Studies indicate that a 5 percent reduction of body water (approximately six cups) may result in a 20 to 30 percent decline in work performance. Athletes guard against water loss for the same reasons, realizing that it takes at least five hours to restore water loss. The athlete most frequently cited as open to the problems of dehydration are wrestlers because they try to "make their weight class" by losing as much water as possible just before the weigh-in.

WATER GAINED   As water is lost in a variety of different ways, it is also gained in a variety of ways. The major source of water are the fluids we drink in the form of beverages and tap water. They represent up to half of that amount. The next important source is solid food. The water content of solid food will vary from virtually none to as much as 95 percent, such as in cucumbers and lettuce.

The body also retrieves water from metabolizing or breaking down fats, carbohydrates, and proteins. The amount of water derived from this process, called metabolic water, makes up about 10 to 20 percent of our total daily needs.

WHO IS AT RISK   Primarily, the people who are at risk of dehydration are people who exert themselves too much and deplete their water supply. The amount of water an athlete loses depends on his or her body weight, the quality of the environment, and the amount of strenuous physical exercise completed. People in relatively good condition lose water but relatively little sodium, which is a related concern of water loss. Those in poor condition, however, will lose water and sodium, and both must be replaced.

The environment can be a factor concerning the risk of water loss. Some credit is given to water for the first successful climb of Mount Everest because the team drank four quarts of water daily to make up for losses due to the increased hyperventilation and dryness of the air. In the past, other climbing teams attempted an assault with water rations of only one quart or less per day.

Other people who may be at some risk of water loss are those who have trouble absorbing water, such as people with chronic diarrhea or poor kidney function, or people who suffer from persistent vomiting.

The experience of thirst is regulated by centers in the hypothalamus, an area of the brain next to the pituitary gland. In a healthy person this urge to drink is a very reliable means of regulating fluid intake. If the hypothalamus is damaged, however, or doesn't function properly, which is rather rare, the thirst mechanism may also malfunction, and severe dehydration can occur.

NOTE   Some health specialists believe that an overlooked area of potential water loss is air travel. The pressurized cabin air is extremely dry and quickly circulated, which vastly accelerates the rate of evaporation. During long flights this environment can pose a problem for some people who may be borderline dehydrated. A traveler can lose as much as a quart of water during a three-and-one-half-hour flight in a standard commercial jet.

TOO MUCH WATER   Someone can actually drink too much water. During a period of intense thirst the body will signal the need for a significant increase in water consumption. If the water intake is very high and is not accompanied by enough sodium (salt) to replace what has been lost, the individual suffers from a condition known as water intoxication. Since the water does not carry an adequate amount of sodium, the cell takes on too much water, a condition called overhydration, which eventually causes the muscles to cramp.

STRATEGIES

FOOD SOURCES   Studies show that among children and teenagers, milk and milk drinks make up an average of 17 ounces per day of their fluid consumption. (Whole milk contains 87 percent water, and skim milk 91 percent.) Among adults and older teenagers the most popular group of beverages was a combination of carbonated and noncarbonated sweet drinks, and tea represented about 12 ounces. Fruit and vegetable juices provide about 7 ounces per day.

Solid foods are the second most important sources of water in our diet. Somewhat surprisingly, a random representative selection of solid foods will contain about 50 percent water. Foods such as cucumbers, lettuce, tomatoes, celery, milk, oranges, oysters, apples, and bananas are made up of at least three-fourths water, and the water content of hamburgers, cooked spaghetti, and raw eggs is more than 50 percent.

Bottled Water: Commercial bottlers will claim that bottled mineral water is safer and more healthful than tap water. The fact of the matter is that all water with the exception of distilled water is mineral water. These natural mineral waters may differ in the amount of dissolved solids or minerals they contain. Many so-called mineral waters contain between 200 milligrams to 400 milligrams of sodium per 8 ounces, which can be a concern for people who must watch their sodium intake.

FOODS THAT AFFECT WATER LOSS   Some foods act as a diuretic, increasing urine flow and depleting water from the body. Because of their caffeine, coffee and tea increase the rate of blood flow through the kidneys and alter the transport of salts and water. Alcohol also acts as a diuretic by depressing the production of ADH (antidiuretic hormone), which causes the kidney to conserve water. If the concentration of substances that must be excreted build up in the kidneys, additional water will be needed. If the water intake does not increase, the water will be drawn from the body fluids or tissues.

Some parents urge their children not to drink water during their meals for fear that it will not only spoil their appetite but will be somehow harmful to proper digestion. In many respects they are right. Water should not be used to wash food down because it might dilute saliva and other digestive juices and discourage children from properly masticating or chewing their food before swallowing. Food should be fully chewed and swallowed before drinking any water or fluid. It is also advised not to drink very cold water during hot weather because it can cause stomach cramping.

TRACE MINERALS

The macrominerals—calcium, phosphorus, magnesium, potassium, sulfur, and chloride—make up nearly 99 percent of the mineral content of the body. The remaining 1 percent are microelements or "trace" elements, but they are no less vital to our health.

We will discuss these trace elements primarily in the order in which they were accepted as essential to human and animal nutrition. The first group was identified as essential before 1960 and consisted of iron, copper, iodine, and manganese. The second group was discovered to be important to good health only in the past thirty years, and they are zinc, fluorine, cobalt, molybdenum, selenium, and chromium. The remaining trace elements presented—nickel, vanadium, silicon, and arsenic—are not uniformly considered essential to human life, but current research reveals that they are essential for animals and possibly some day research may point to their necessity to human life as well. It is interesting to note that since 1979 two trace elements—molybdenum and selenium—that were considered necessary only for animals were reclassified as essential to human life as a result of new studies.

Finally, three other trace elements present in foods—tin, lead, and boron—are mentioned at the close of this section since current studies have revealed some interesting possibilities as to their nutritional value.

IRON

DESCRIPTION

The most important function of iron is in the formation of hemoglobin. Hemoglobin transports oxygen in the blood from the lungs to the tissues. Iron is also necessary for the formation of myoglobin, an iron-containing compound that is responsible for providing oxygen to muscle tissue, which is required for muscle contraction. Iron is found in the enzymes that promote protein metabolism, and it works with other nutrients to improve respiratory action. Iron also increases the general resistance to stress and disease.

FOOD SOURCES

Excellent sources: pork, lamb, calf's liver, beef, chicken, raisins, soybeans, fried figs, and baked beans
Good sources: molasses (blackstrap), cooked peas, dried apricots, whole-wheat cereals, spinach, and lima beans

HIGH-RISK GROUPS FOR POSSIBLE DEFICIENCY

- pregnant or breast-feeding women
- women of child-bearing age
- people suffering from bulimia (persistent vomiting)
- people on a severe low-calorie diet
- strict vegetarians (vegans)
- woman who suffer from heavy menstrual bleeding
- people with bleeding hemorrhoids
- people who chronically use aspirin
- people with celiac disease
- people over the age of 60
- people recovering from gastrointestinal surgery or severe burns
- athletes or workers who participate in strenuous activity
- people who use prescription drugs that cause microscopic gastric bleeding, such as Nalidixic Acid (NegGram), and Indomethacin (Indocin)

- people who use drugs that cause malabsorption of iron such as Neomycin Sulfate and Tetracycline, and Para-Aminosalicylic Acid, Allopurinal (Lopurin and Zyloprim), and Clofibrate (Atromid-S)
- people who regularly take caffeine-containing drugs
- people who take drugs that retard gastric acid secretion, such as Cimetidine (Tagamet)
- people who use olive oil as a laxative

RECOMMENDED DOSAGE

GROUP	MG	GROUP	MG
Pregnant women	30	Children 7–10	10
Lactating women	30	Young women 11–18	18
Infants 0–0.5	10	19–22	18
0.5–1	15	Young men 11–18	18
Children 1–3	15	19–22	10
4–6	10	Adult women 23–50	15
		51 +	10
		Adult men 23–50	10
		51 +	10

* Pregnant women in their third trimester require more iron than is generally available in the average diet. It is therefore recommended that they take 30 milligrams of ferrous sulfate (which is equivalent to 6 mg. of iron). Women who are breast-feeding need to replace their iron stores depleted by the pregnancy.)

UPPER LIMITS OF REGULAR DIETARY SUPPLEMENT USE

Children under 4 years of age: 15 mg
Adults and children 4 or more years of age: 27 mg
Pregnant or lactating women: 60 mg

TOXIC LEVELS

Have not been established.

BENEFITS

TREATING DEFICIENCY SYMPTOMS

MILD DEFICIENCY
- fatigue
- listlessness
- irritability
- loss of appetite

GROSS DEFICIENCY
- paleness of skin
- coldness and tingling of hands and feet
- shortness of breath
- rapid heart rate

OTHER POSSIBLE BENEFITS

- reduces blood fat levels

UNPROVEN BENEFITS (UNRELATED TO DEFICIENCY SYMPTOMS)

- controls alcoholism
- increases immunity
- treatment of leukemia
- anti-aging properties

TOXIC SYMPTOMS
Nausea, intestinal pains, bloody diarrhea, and vomiting with blood.

DISCOVERY In 1684 Robert Boyle, the great British physicist and chemist, noted that the burnt ash of blood was curiously brick red. The ash was in fact iron, and less than forty years later it was conclusively established that iron was a constituent of body tissue and present in human blood; however, virtually everything else we know about iron has been the work of twentieth-century modern chemistry. In this century we have learned that dietary iron provides many varied and extremely important functions.

DIFFERENT KINDS OF IRON Not all dietary iron is the same. Iron appears in our food in two different forms—heme iron and nonheme (ionic) iron. About 40 percent of the iron in meat is part of the hemoglobin molecule known as heme iron. All other dietary iron from plant food and from the iron-containing parts of animal tissues other than heme, is nonheme iron.

The significant difference between these two forms of dietary iron is that heme iron in meat protein is 15 to 35 percent available, which means that we absorb about one-third of it. That is not bad in light of the fact that we absorb only 3 to 10 percent of nonheme iron.

ABSORPTION We don't absorb every bit of every nutrient —vitamin or mineral—we consume. Their absorption depends upon a number of factors, including the chemical makeup of the nutrient itself.

Generally, the maximum absorption of iron is about 40 percent for an adult. (Infants can absorb as much as 50 percent of the iron they receive from their mother's milk.) One factor that can improve the absorption of iron is normal acid levels in the stomach. Certain acidic foods such as orange juice can increase the absorption of nonheme iron by as much as three times. In addition to citric acid, the presence of vitamin C also aids absorption, and a well-balanced diet with plenty of meat protein is yet another aid to iron absorption.

Foods that Lower Iron Absorption: Phytic acid, which is found especially in bran, reduces absorption by forming insoluble compounds with iron. (It does the same with calcium.) This accounts for the poor absorption of iron from whole wheat (also about 2 to 5 percent) and provides some explanation as to why there is a high incidence of iron-deficient anemia in countries that rely upon whole wheat for their major source of carbohydrates.

Foods containing tannins (for example, commercial black tea), foods that contribute oxalates (for example, chocolate, blueberries, and summer squash), foods rich in phosphates (for example, cheese), and coffee (which contains a substance called *polyphenol*) all decrease iron absorption. Furthermore, foods that contain zinc salts and foods high in fiber, especially the fiber found in corn and wheat, can also inhibit iron absorption.

ROLE   Two-thirds of the iron in the body is used to transport oxygen, to take it from the lungs and later to form with other substances. This is accomplished through the means of an iron-containing protein in the red blood cell called a hemoglobin (in Latin *hemo* means blood and *globus* means world). Iron is also involved with ridding the body of carbon dioxide since the hemoglobin also picks up the carbon dioxide from the cell and carries it to the lungs to be expelled. With the help of another iron-containing compound, myoglobin (in Greek *mys* means muscle), much needed oxygen is carried to the cells of the muscles.

As a part of a hormone called erythropoietin, iron is essential to red blood cell production, and it is a party to many other oxygen exchanges in cell tissue. Iron is present in the enzymes that help metabolize protein, and it works with other nutrients to improve respiratory action.

Iron is important in functions such as the production of collagen, which is the protein that forms the matrix or mortar for the bone (see Calcium, page 148), the production of antibodies, the detoxification of drugs in the liver, the synthesis of nucleic acids, the removal of fats from the blood, and the conversion of beta-carotene to vitamin A (see Vitamin A, page 56).

The fact that a deficiency of iron reduces the production of iron-containing enzymes and other immune substances that are necessary to fight infectious organisms strongly suggests that iron is an integral part of any defense against infections. Further evidence for this claim is found in the fact that iron in breast milk binds with an infectious organism found in the gastrointestinal tract of infants (E. coli) that prevents the growth of a potentially serious intestinal infection.

NOTE   Many pediatricians and nutritionists believe that human milk does not supply adequate amounts of iron for the newborn. This is not necessarily worrisome because most breast-fed infants do not generally develop any iron-deficient symptoms since nearly half of all the iron in breast milk is absorbed by the infant and most babies are born with a three- to six-month supply. On the other hand, the argument that infants should receive some iron supplementation over the course of the first year rests on the fact that most calculations of infant needs for this period exceed what is available in normal human milk and what is held in reserve by the infant. For these reasons, the Academy of Pediatrics recommends that infants be given iron-fortified milk during the first year of life.

CONSERVATION   The body is very prudent in its conservation of dietary iron, especially in the stores of iron found in the billions of red blood cells. (There is probably 4.5 to 5 million red blood cells per cubic millimeter and a total of one teaspoon of iron in the entire body.) When a red blood cell dies and disintegrates, the hemoglobin divides into an iron-containing dark brown substance—oxidized heme—and a pigment called bilirubin. Much of this oxidized iron is recovered (along with the bilirubin) and used to form new red blood cells; the unused excess is secreted in liver bile and passed out in the feces. The excreted iron is what gives color to feces.

PROBLEMS OF TOO LITTLE Since the body tenaciously hangs on to its iron, a deficiency generally occurs only when the demand is up, such as during growth periods, during a pregnancy, and when there is a loss of blood. Nevertheless, an iron deficiency may be the most common form of malnutrition in the world. In this country, folic acid and vitamin B12 are common deficiencies that lead to anemia, but iron-deficiency anemia is by far the most common nutrient deficiency disease, and it primarily affects women.

The most common symptoms of iron deficiency is anemia. A lack of iron reduces the oxygen-carrying capacity of the blood, which directly affects the performance of muscle and tissue throughout the body. Consequently, someone suffering from a lack of adequate iron will easily tire and may also complain of a general listlessnes, irritability, and a lack of interest in food. If the deficiency becomes severe, it may produce extremely pale skin and lips, a coldness and tingling in the hands and feet, and a shortness of breath. In some cases the individual may have a persistently rapid heart rate.

Even if anemia is not present, growth periods usually demand an increase in iron. An inadequate iron supply, especially among teenage children whose iron needs are relatively high, might produce symptoms such as poor stamina, poor school performance, or an increase in the number of infections. Adults may experience trouble with digestion and changes in the tissues inside the mouth or esophagus. Another sign of poor iron stores is thin, brittle, very flat, or spoon-shaped fingernails.

WHO IS AT RISK Studies suggest that 10 percent of all women suffer from an iron deficiency, and as many as one out of every three women has low iron stores.

One group that researchers believe is widely iron deficient and experiences nutritional anemia as well are adolescent girls. The problem grows out of the fact that their iron intake cannot match their needs due to menstrual losses and the increased demands of adolescent growth. The fact is that blood loss through menstruation continues to be a source of iron depletion for all women throughout their lives. The average woman loses about 15 to 20 milligrams of iron each menstrual period, but there is considerable variation among individual women. Some studies found that as many as 10 percent of the women tested lost 40 milligrams of iron per period. On a daily basis this loss would call for an additional 14 milligrams of iron or a total daily need of 24 milligrams. The choice of contraception methods may also affect the extent of blood loss in some women. Even bleeding hemorrhoids can increase the risk of an iron deficiency.

People who take aspirin on a daily basis, such as arthritis patients, are at risk because aspirin can cause microscopic bleeding and a subsequent loss of iron. As many as 70 percent of those who take 1 to 3 grams of aspirin per day develop gastrointestinal bleeding. The most characteristic sign of this condition is black and tarry stools.

The elderly are also prone to iron deficiencies because they produce less hydrochloric acid in their later years, which is necessary for successful iron absorption.

Disorders such as bulimia in which the patient goes on an eating binge and then induces vomiting can be the cause of an iron deficiency because the food has not been allowed to digest properly. People on a severe low-calorie diet are at risk, and this applies especially to strict vegetarians (vegans) because their diet is low in iron; also, much of the iron in their diet may be nonheme, which is not readily absorbed. A lack of iron shows up also in those who have general absorption problems, such as celiac disease, and those who recently have had intestinal surgery.

TOO MUCH IRON   Toxic levels of iron can be reached if iron supplements are used excessively. The safe range could be as much as ten to thirty times the allowance, but only for a short period—one to two weeks. Over longer periods even smaller doses can cause toxic symptoms such as vomiting blood, bloody diarrhea, nausea, and acute abdominal pain. In some cases excessive iron can cause the skin to look bronzed.

Another consideration is the amount of a single dose. Some people find they have a low tolerance for doses of highly ionizable iron, such as ferrous sulfate, if taken in amounts of 200 milligrams or more a day. In some cases doses of 200 milligrams have produced poisoning in young children. Before you take iron supplements that greatly exceed RDA levels, consult a physician.

STRATEGIES

FOOD SOURCES   The more readily absorbed heme iron plays a crucial role in our diet. Specifically, this is one of the reasons pork, lamb, calf's liver, beef, chicken, and fish are particularly nutritious.

In fact, it is believed that up to one-third of our daily iron needs come from these sources. Some other good nonheme iron sources are raisins, soybeans, fried figs, baked beans, molasses (blackstrap), cooked peas, dried apricots, whole-wheat cereals, spinach, and lima beans.

Cereals, flour, and some breads are enriched with iron, though some nutritionists fear that these enriched foods could lead to iron overload and create possible liver, heart, and pancreatic damage in some people, especially men who eat iron-rich diets. This concern seems misplaced since iron deficiencies, however modest, are widespread, and red meat consumption is on the decline in this country.

The average diet contributes iron in approximately the following proportions: 29 percent from meat, poultry and fish; flour and cereal products provide another 29 percent; eggs yield 5 percent; dairy products (except butter which has no iron) contribute 2.5 percent; fruits offer a little more than 4 percent, as do sweet and white potatoes; 1.5 percent comes from dark green and deep yellow vegetables, while other vegetables such as tomatoes offer 9 percent; dry beans and peas, nuts, soy flour, and grits produce 7 percent; and sweeteners, including sugars, contribute about 7 percent; and the balance from miscellaneous foods is 2 percent.

FOOD PREPARATION   Iron is lost in food preparation principally when the cooking water is discarded. A second loss occurs when food is peeled and discarded since iron is concentrated near the surface of these foods. Losses can be minimized by cooking your food at lower temperatures, in less water (steaming is preferable), and in larger pieces. The use of the water in gravies or soup stock salvages much of the iron loss.

DRUG INTERACTIONS   Allopurinol (Lopurin and Zyloprim), drugs prescribed for the treatment of gout, impair the absorption of iron. The persistent use of aspirin causes microscopic bleeding that will lead to a subsequent iron loss. Indomethacin (Indocin), an anti-inflammatory drug, also causes gastric irritation and microscopic bleeding, which means more iron loss.

Caffeine, especially as a drug (for example, Dexatrim and Amaphen with Codeine), can impair iron absorption. Coffee use will only marginally affect iron loss.

Because Cimetidine (Tagament) inhibits the secretion of gastric acid, it negatively affects iron which needs acid for its absorption, especially the nonheme iron from vegetables. People with low iron stores could conceivably develop a deficiency with the use of this drug.

Clofibrate (Atromid-S), which is a cholesterol-reducing drug, creates malabsorption problems for both vitamin B12 and iron.

The absorption of iron is adversely affected when taken with antacids or foods rich in phosphates (for example, cheese) and high fiber (bran) foods. Vitamin C is helpful to iron absorption, but vitamin E will decrease its effectiveness in the body. It is advised, therefore, to take vitamin C or foods rich in ascorbic acid and avoid vitamin E supplements while taking iron supplements, particularly if you are iron deficient.

The antibiotic Nalidixic Acid (NegGram) is a gastric irritant that often causes gastric bleeding and iron losses. Long-term use of the antibiotic Neomycin Sulfate can cause problems for iron since it impairs the absorption of most nutrients. Tetracycline, another antibiotic, impairs iron absorption, but iron supplements can impair the absorption of tetracycline. Para-Aminosalicylic Acid, an antitubercular drug, also creates a malabsorption problem for iron.

Those people who choose to use olive oil as a laxative may have a problem since the oil interferes with the general absorption of most nutrients. (The quantities used in cooking do not pose any problem.)

COPPER

DESCRIPTION

Because copper is a trace element that aids in the absorption of iron, it directly affects the formation of hemoglobin, which is the oxygen-carrying protein of the red blood cell. Copper is involved in the conversion of an amino acid that colors hair and skin, and it is required in the production of substances that form a protective shield around nerve fibers. Copper also helps the body oxidize vitamin C and is necessary for proper bone growth.

FOOD SOURCES

Excellent sources: liver and kidney meats, shellfish (especially oysters and crab), nuts, and seeds
Good sources: wheat, corn, dried beans, legumes, and cocoa

HIGH-RISK GROUPS FOR POSSIBLE DEFICIENCY

- people on a severe low-calorie diet
- people over 60 years of age
- pregnant or breast-feeding women
- alcoholics
- people suffering from chronic diarrhea
- people suffering from kidney disease
- infants who receive only cow's milk without supplements
- people recovering from gastrointestinal surgery

RECOMMENDED DOSAGE

GROUP	MG	GROUP	MG
Pregnant women	2.0–3.0	Children 7–10	2.0–2.5
Lactating women	2.0–3.0	Adolescents 11–18	2.0–3.0
Infants 0–0.5	0.5–0.7	Adults 18 +	2.0–3.0
0.5–1	0.7–1.0		
Children 1–3	1.0–1.5		
4–6	1.5–2.0		

UPPER LIMITS FOR DIETARY SUPPLEMENT USE

Children under 4 years of age:	12.0 mg
Adults and children 4 or more years of age:	22.5 mg
Pregnant or lactating women:	4.0 mg

BENEFITS

TREATING DEFICIENCY SYMPTOMS
- anemia
- iron deficiency treatments

OTHER POSSIBLE BENEFITS
- preventing osteoporosis

UNPROVEN BENEFITS (UNRELATED TO DEFICIENCY SYMPTOMS)

- prevention and treatment of arthritis
- prevents hair loss
- treats leukemia

TOXIC SYMPTOMS

Nausea, vomiting, muscle aches, and abdominal pain.

DISCOVERY In 1924 researchers at the University of Wisconsin who were involved in a study to determine what nutritional factors influenced the formation of hemoglobin (red blood cells) were surprised to learn that test animals were not capable of utilizing the iron in their diet to produce hemoglobin. However, when they were fed relatively small amounts of dried kidney and liver as part of their regular diet, the animals were able to make hemoglobin.

The biochemists who studied the ash from the dried kidney and liver assumed that the pale blue color was from copper salts. They therefore added copper sulfate to the diet of the test animals, and the animals immediately began to produce hemoglobin. This was the first conclusive evidence that copper was essential in the formation of hemoglobin.

ROLE Iron relies on copper to perform many of its functions. Copper stimulates the synthesis of the heme or iron of the hemoglobin molecule, and it is associated with the release of stored iron from the liver. It also plays a role in the oxidation of iron in the body. As a result, copper actually helps prevent iron-deficiency anemia because it directly affects the very utilization of the mineral.

Copper is needed to form the shield called *myelin* that surrounds the nerve fibers and protects them. It also helps release iron for the synthesis of hemoglobin and the metabolism of glucose; it maintains enzymes (along with vitamin C) that produce collagen, which is responsible for healthy bones; and through yet other enzymes, it is responsible for melanin, which is the dark pigment of the hair and skin.

PROBLEMS OF TOO LITTLE   Generally, copper deficiencies occur only among infants, either because of a genetic defect or because their diet during ages six to twelve months failed to provide adequate amounts of copper. The symptoms associated with a copper deficiency are retarded growth, some scurvylike symptoms (skin disorders), fluctuating temperature, anemia, and coarse hair like steel wool.

WHO IS AT RISK   This is a rare deficiency among humans. When it is seen, it is usually found in infants less than a year old who have been fed only cow's milk and have had diarrhea. Infants are born with enough copper to last three to six months, but if their diet is copper deficient, they can develop deficiency symptoms during the second six months of their life. It is also possible that copper-deficient infants are unable to reabsorb the copper that is already in their body.

Adults seldom see a copper deficiency. Pregnant and lactating women have a known increased need for copper, but even then it is not enough to cause a deficiency.

ABSORPTION   As much as 50 percent of the copper in our food is absorbed. Absorption can be impaired, however, by consuming high levels of zinc salts and by excessive antacid use. At least one case has been reported of a woman developing a copper deficiency while taking megadoses of antacid, despite the fact that she consumed an otherwise normal diet.

TOO MUCH   There is no evidence of copper toxicity due to the consumption of a normal diet or to environmental contamination. However, Wilson's disease is a rare chronic metabolic disorder in which the body is unable to excrete very much copper, and in these cases, toxic amounts of copper can accumulate in the liver, brain, kidneys, and eyes.

STRATEGIES

FOOD SOURCES   Minute amounts of copper appear in many foods, with the average diet containing from 2 to 5 milligrams per day. The best sources are calf's liver, shellfish (especially oysters and canned crab), nuts, seeds (especially Brazil and hickory nuts, sesame and sunflower seeds), dry beans (especially navy, soy, kidney, and limas), molasses, cocoa, chocolate, caffeine-free ground coffee, tea, and dried yeast.

FOOD PREPARATION   Copper is inadvertently added to food in processing, as is iodine. Iodine-containing compounds used in sanitizing the processing equipment in milk production add iodine. In the same manner, copper is unintentionally added to milk as the milk passes over copper rollers during the pasteurization process. Minute amounts of copper appear in those foods that are prepared in copper pans and in the drinking water of homes with copper plumbing.

DRUG INTERACTIONS   The use of zinc supplements could conceivably lead to a copper deficiency. Furthermore, megadoses of vitamin C will decrease copper absorption.

IODINE

DESCRIPTION

Iodine is a "trace" mineral, or micronutrient, that is critical to the functioning of the thyroid gland. Without the presence of iodine, the gland would be unable to produce the hormones that regulate the body's production of energy, its growth and development. Iodine also affects the growth of hair, nails, and teeth, and the absorption of carbohydrates from the intestine. Vitamin A depends on iodine, too.

FOOD SOURCES

Excellent sources: (other than iodized salt): dairy products, seafood, and poultry

Good sources: bread and cereal products, candy, cake mixes, sugared breakfast cereals, and confectionary products

HIGH-RISK GROUPS FOR POSSIBLE DEFICIENCY

- people on a severe low-calorie diet
- people who live where the soil or water is poor in iodine
- people whose diet is dominated by goitrogen-containing foods

RECOMMENDED DOSAGE

GROUP	MCG	GROUP	MCG
Pregnant women	175	Children 7–10	120
Lactating women	200	Young Women 11–22	150
Infants 0–0.6	40	Adult women 23 +	150
0.6–1	50	Young Men 11–22	150
Children 1–3	70	Adult Men 23+	150
4–6	90		

UPPER LIMITS FOR REGULAR DIETARY SUPPLEMENT USE

Children under 4 years of age: 105 mcg

Adults and children 4 or more years of age: 225 mcg

Pregnant or lactating women: 300 mcg

BENEFITS

TREATING DEFICIENCY SYMPTOMS
- goiters (an enlarged thyroid gland)
- dull hair, weak nails, and skin disorders

OTHER POSSIBLE BENEFITS
- prevents high cholesterol levels

UNPROVEN BENEFITS (UNRELATED TO DEFICIENCY SYMPTOMS)

- treats arthritis
- treats angina pectoris

- cures anemia

TOXIC SYMPTOMS

Bloody or tarry black stool (caused by bleeding), irregular heartbeat, mental confusion.

DISCOVERY   The history of our understanding of dietary iodine is related to the history of a disease caused by its deficiency: goiters. Goiters is an easily identified disease since it produces a swollen thyroid gland that appears as an evident enlargement at the base of the neck.

It is believed that as long ago as 3000 B.C. in China, goiters were treated effectively by feeding seaweed or burnt sponges to those affected. In 1811 a French chemist, Bernard Courtois, was in the business of making gunpowder, which is potassium nitrate. While burning seaweed for its potassium ash, he noticed that the seaweed gave off a violet-colored vapor, and when he condensed it, the vapor formed dark lustrous crystals. When the English chemist Sir Humphry Davy duplicated this experiment, he suggested calling this new element *iodine,* a word formed from the Greek *ioeides,* which means violet-colored. Within ten years a Swiss physician, J. R. Coindet, produced the conclusive evidence that established iodine as the curative substance that made seaweed and burnt sponge so effective in the treatment of goiters.

In the latter part of the nineteenth century, chemists and physicians began to see more clearly the connection between iodine and goiters and suspected that goiters may be a dietary deficiency disease. Proof of this claim was established in 1895 when it was determined that iodine was a normal constituent of the thyroid gland. Following this discovery, it was widely assumed that any endemic or widespread occurrence of goiters was the result of poor levels of iodine in the diet and that iodine therapy would be an effective treatment for the disease.

In this country an outbreak of goiters in the state of Ohio led to the first community-organized treatment for goiters. Specifically, iodine tablets were added to the Ohio water supply twice a year from 1916 to 1920, and they dramatically reduced the incidence of goiters. Another experiment involved feeding iodized salt to dairy cows to improve the iodine contents of their milk. These efforts and others like them were successful, but it was the mandating and distribution of iodized salt that proved to be the most effective means of protecting a majority of the population from iodine deficiencies.

ROLE   Iodine is found in the thyroid gland where it is an essential constituent of thyroid hormone, *thyroxin*. The principal function of iodine-containing hormone is to regulate the metabolism in the cells, which means the production of energy in the cells and their growth and development. Because iodine is central to the production and effectiveness of other hormones, it could be said that iodine is equally essential to their vital functions; for example, thyroid hormones play a role in neurological functions, including an effect on the speech center of the brain, and they also affect the health of hair, nails, and teeth.

The absorption of carbohydrates from the intestine is made more efficient when thyroxin levels are normal, and thyroxin also affects blood cholesterol levels.

Finally, the body relies on iodine to convert carotene to an active form of vitamin A, and iodine is also necessary for the synthesis of protein.

PROBLEMS OF TOO LITTLE   Too little iodine produces hypothyroidism and goiters, a condition in which the thyroid gland in the neck becomes enlarged as a result of insufficient iodine. (The name goiter is derived from the Latin word for throat, *guttur*). Because of a deficiency of iodine in their mothers during the first three months of pregnancy or before conception, some children develop cretinism, a disastrous malady in which the children are usually undersized, mentally slow, and hearing impaired, and usually have relatively short life spans.

WHO IS AT RISK   The incidence of goiters is six times higher among females, especially adolescent girls and pregnant women.

TOO MUCH   This is a rare problem because the dietary levels of iodine are well below toxic levels. It can be a problem for thyroid-sensitive people who treat themselves with compounds of iodide or concentrates of dried seaweed.

STRATEGIES

FOOD SOURCES   The amount of iodine in our food varies, depending on the amount in the soil and water in which the food was grown. The iodine content of seawater (and seafood) is from ten to one hundred times greater than that of fresh water (and freshwater fish).

Even within fresh waters, the iodine of glacial rivers and lakes are lower than others that are not glacial in origin. Iodine content of soil also varies throughout the country; for example, the soil of Louisiana is richer in iodine than that of Oklahoma, while Florida's is much poorer than that of Oklahoma.

In addition to the soil affecting the iodine content of certain foods, iodine-containing compounds used in sanitizing processing equipment make milk and dairy products good food sources of iodine. Iodate dough conditioners used in bread-making and iodine-containing food coloring agents also make significant contributions to our dietary iodine. But the major contribution of iodine to our diet comes from the presence and use of iodized salt.

In addition to seafood, especially lobster, shrimp, and oysters, other good sources of iodine are cake mixes, confectionary products, and many candies.

The federal government states that the labeling of salt must indicate whether it includes "iodine, an essential nutrient." If it does not include iodine, the salt must state "This product does not contain iodine." Contrary to public opinion, sea salt is not necessarily a good source of iodine because iodine converts to vapor as the salt dries. For foods that impair iodine absorption, see the table of Goitrogen-Rich Foods, page 249.

Without considering the addition of table salt, the average adult diet contains salt in these proportions: dairy products provide 56 percent; cereal and grain products, 16 percent; meat, fish, and poultry contain about 11 percent; sugars about 10 percent; beverages (and this includes drinking water) about 4 percent; and all other foods, including vegetables and fruits, a little more than 3 percent.

DRUG INTERACTIONS Thiazides, which are strong diuretics, can increase the risk of hypothyroidism for those who are marginally deficient in iodine. The drug poses this kind of problem because it dramatically increases iodine excretion.

MANGANESE

DESCRIPTION
Manganese, another trace element, plays a role in many enzymes and thereby is involved in such activities as the utilization of choline, biotin, thiamine, and ascorbic acid. It is essential to the synthesis of fatty acids and cholesterol and the metabolism of complex carbohydrates and fat production. It also is important to the nervous system and in the maintenance of sex hormones.

FOOD SOURCES
Excellent sources: whole-grain cereals (especially buckwheat and oatmeals), egg yolks, bananas, nuts (especially hazelnuts, pecans, and chestnuts), and seeds
Good sources: dried beans, peas, spinach, blackberries, avocados, and ginger

HIGH-RISK GROUPS FOR POSSIBLE DEFICIENCY
None.

RECOMMENDED DOSAGE

GROUP	MG	GROUP	MG
Infants 0–0.6	0.5–0.7	Children 7–10	2.0–3.0
0.6–1	0.7–1.0	Children and adults 11 +	2.5–5.0
Children 1–3	1.0–1.5		
4–6	1.5–2.0		

UPPER LIMITS OF REGULAR DIETARY SUPPLEMENT USE
The provisional maximum intakes have not been determined, but intakes that are less than .7 milligrams are considered inadequate.

TOXIC LEVELS
Have not been established.

BENEFITS

TREATING DEFICIENCY SYMPTOMS
No deficiency has been demonstrated in humans. Deficiency symptoms have occurred only in experimental conditions.

- (Possible) failure to grow in children
- (Possible) reproductive disorder

UNPROVEN BENEFITS (UNRELATED TO DEFICIENCY SYMPTOMS)

- treats asthma
- cures infertility
- treats diabetes
- anti-aging substance

TOXIC SYMPTOMS
Insomnia, depression, impotence, delusions, and nerve degeneration, causing Parkinson's disease-like symptoms.

ROLE Manganese has been confused, understandably, with another metal element, magnesium. Not only are their names similar but they are derived from the same name, *magnesium alba*. (Magnesium takes its name from Magnesia, a region in ancient Thessaly (Greece) where the white mineral—magnesia salt—was first discovered.) Though two different elements with different functions in the body, they are both involved in bone formation.

The principal functions of manganese may be in the formation of bone structure, for reproduction, and for normal functioning of the nervous system. Because it is part of the enzyme system, it is connected with numerous metabolic activities (more than most trace elements) such as the metabolism of fatty acids, the synthesis of cholesterol and complex carbohydrates, the utilization of glucose, the development of a normal pancreas, muscle contraction, and the prevention of skeletal defects and sterility.

PROBLEMS OF TOO LITTLE There is no conclusive evidence of a human deficiency of manganese. Under laboratory conditions manganese deficiencies have caused a failure of growth in young animals and an inability to reproduce in female animals. Poultry producers have reported manganese deficiencies that have caused deformed legs among fowl. Both a deficiency and an excess of manganese also adversely affects the brain and nervous systems of the animals.

Though manganese deficiencies are very unlikely, it should be mentioned that high intakes of iron and calcium will decrease manganese absorption, whereas high levels of dietary protein protect against malabsorption.

STRATEGIES

FOOD SOURCES Manganese is widely distributed throughout many foods, especially those of plant origin. Buckwheat, oatmeal, and other whole-grain cereals are rich in manganese, and nuts such as hazelnuts, pecans, and chestnuts are good sources. Vegetables such as dried beans, peas, and spinach are also good sources, as are some fruits such as bananas and blackberries. Meats, poultry, and dairy products contribute a little, and seafood and fish have the lowest amounts of manganese. The amount of manganese present in any food will depend on the soil in which it was grown or fed.

Tea is an extremely good source. In fact, it is thought that it contributes as much as 2.3 milligrams per day in the average British diet.

FOOD PREPARATION Little or no manganese is lost in normal cooking procedures, but some is lost in the refining of some foods.

DRUG INTERACTIONS None.

ZINC

DESCRIPTION

Zinc is a constituent of many enzymes that are involved with digestion and metabolism. It favorably affects the absorption of vitamin A, it is a part of insulin, and it is needed to break down alcohol. Zinc is critical to removing carbon dioxide from the cells and is essential to the growth and development of the reproductive organs and functioning of the prostate gland. It also appears to be of value in healing wounds and burns.

FOOD SOURCES

Excellent sources: seafood (especially canned tuna, sardines, and oysters), lamb chops, lean beef (especially liver), and pork

Good sources: whole-wheat grains, root vegetables (especially white turnips), nuts (especially Brazil nuts and pecans), and popcorn

HIGH-RISK GROUPS FOR POSSIBLE DEFICIENCY

- people on a severe low-calorie diet
- pregnant and breast-feeding women
- preschool children
- people over the age of 60
- alcoholics
- people recovering from gastrointestinal surgery or severe burns
- people who use diuretics regularly

RECOMMENDED DOSAGE

GROUP	MG	GROUP	MG
Pregnant women	20	Children 7–10	10
Lactating women	25	Young women 11–22	15
Infants 0–0.5	3	Adult women 23 +	15
0.5–1	5	Young men 11–22	15
Children 1–3	10	Adult men 23 +	15
4–6			

UPPER LIMITS FOR REGULAR DIETARY SUPPLEMENT USE
Children under 4 years of age: 5 mg
Adult and children 4 or more years of age: 20mg
Pregnant or lactating women: 30 mg

TOXIC LEVELS
Have not been established.

BENEFITS
TREATING DEFICIENCY SYMPTOMS
- loss of appetite
- poor growth
- acne and congenital skin disorders
- treats loss of taste
- dental decay

OTHER POSSIBLE BENEFITS
- strengthening of the immune system
- favorably affects learning behaviors

UNPROVEN BENEFITS (UNRELATED TO DEFICIENCY SYMPTOMS)
- treatment of schizophrenia
- treatment of diabetes
- prevention of infertility
- prevention and treatment of acne

TOXIC SYMPTOMS
Nausea, bloating, cramps, diarrhea, and fever.

DISCOVERY In the middle of the nineteenth century biochemists were coming to believe that organic compounds could be formed with metals for some use in the body. It was not until the 1930s, however, at the University of Wisconsin that clear-cut proof was established concerning the nutritional value of zinc and its essential need in the diet of mammals.

For many years, symptoms such as retarded growth and delayed sexual maturation were associated with a lack of dietary zinc in humans. In 1961 evidence of a zinc deficiency in humans was proven, and in 1974 the Food and Nutrition Board included zinc among the nutrients with recommended dietary allowances (RDA).

ROLE Zinc is a constituent of as many as forty enzymes, many that are involved in digestion and metabolism. It is central to the transportation and removal of carbon dioxide from the cells through the bloodstream and to the lungs, and it is essential for respiration. It also favorably affects the absorption of vitamin A, and it is required to break down alcohol.

Some of the many important functions in which zinc plays a role are normal growth (it is clearly associated with the prevention of dwarfism), the prevention of infections, the healing of tissue and wounds, reproduction and the health of reproductive organs, functioning of the prostate gland, and taste perception.

PROBLEMS OF TOO LITTLE A lack of zinc can cause a number of abnormalities in the unborn child, especially smaller babies, and more severe deficiencies can cause cleft palates and brain disorders. Young men who are zinc deficient show evidence of poor sperm production and reduced testosterone, the male hormone that stimulates and promotes the growth of secondary sexual characteristics and the production of sperm.

Recent studies have pointed to the possibility that zinc deficiencies could adversely affect learning behavior and abilities, as well as cause lethargy, amnesia, and mental retardation. Zinc has been found to be one of the most important nutrients for a proper functioning immune system, and if zinc intake is poor, bacterial and viral infections seem to be more severe.

ZINC SUPPLEMENTS There is no evidence that consuming large amounts of zinc supplements will improve immunity or prevent diseases or assure a child of maximum growth potential. These and other zinc-related disorders can be prevented by eating the recommended dietary allowance of zinc per day.

Research on the possible relationship between zinc and cancer is still inconclusive, according to the National Academy of Science. The relation of zinc to our ability to taste or smell is also highly controversial and inconclusive. If a zinc deficiency is not the cause of a lack of taste, zinc supplements will not cure the problem.

A zinc deficiency is only one of several underlying problems that could cause skin disorders. A zinc deficiency can nevertheless produce skin rashes, an acnelike disorder, and they can appear on other parts of the body while the face remains clear. Since a lack of zinc is not associated with common teenage acne, zinc treatments are totally inappropriate.

It is suspected that a lack of zinc may also impair the metabolism of vitamin A, whose deficiency can cause night blindness (an inability to adjust vision to dim light).

WHO IS AT RISK Until recently it was thought that zinc deficiencies were rare in this country, but recent studies citing the fact of delayed healing of wounds and poor growth performance among some children, which are signs of a possible zinc deficiency, suggest that zinc intakes may be lower than previously thought. This does not mean that any one group is at risk of a deficiency, but children entering their principal growth periods, pregnant or lactating women, and women whose menstrual losses are heavy may experience zinc shortages.

Formula-fed babies may also require more because the zinc in cow's milk is less available than in human milk.

People who have any difficulty absorbing zinc, such as those who are recovering from gastrointestinal surgery, may be at risk as well as those who regularly take diuretics.

TOO MUCH Long-term studies are incomplete as to the possible harm from megadoses of zinc supplements, but there is no reason to take more than 30 milligrams of zinc and certainly not over an extended period. One disturbing study revealed that a number of otherwise healthy men who took over 400 milligrams of zinc sulfate developed hardening of the arteries.

HAIR ANALYSIS A number of nutritionists use hair samples as a means for analyzing mineral status. This is a legitimate technique, but it is not without its flaws. In theory, levels of trace elements in hair should reflect levels of body stores, but in practice mineral status should not be determined without some other confirming evidence. Hair can become contaminated by trace elements from shampoos, hair lotions, bleaches, dyes, and other environmental sources. Consequently, cadmium, lead, and mercury levels found in the hair should not be considered a reflection of the same levels of contamination in the body.

STRATEGIES

FOOD SOURCES Zinc appears in almost all foods, but not all foods are rich in this trace mineral. Seafood, meat, whole grains, and nuts are good to excellent sources of zinc, while fruits, vegetables, white flour, and processed food are relatively poor. Milk products, eggs, sweet potatoes, and white turnips are among some of the better sources.

The zinc from plant foods is not as well absorbed as the zinc found in animal foods. (The animal already has absorbed the zinc, making it more available to humans.) Animal food probably provides as much as 70 percent of our dietary zinc needs.

FOOD PREPARATION Processing foods can cause a loss of zinc in some food. Milling, for example, may cause as much as 80 percent of the zinc to be lost. (The husks lost in the milling are fed to the animals which reintroduces the lost zinc to the food cycle.) Very little zinc is lost in home food preparation because, like all minerals and unlike most vitamins, zinc is not heat sensitive.

FLUORINE

DESCRIPTION
Fluorine is found primarily in the skeleton and bones of the body, and is found in the body in compounds called fluorides. It protects against calcium loss during menopause, and it helps to reduce the formation of acid in the mouth caused by carbohydrates, reducing the likelihood of tooth enamel decay.

FOOD SOURCES
Note: The use of fluoridated water or soil rich in fluorides will greatly influence the fluorine content of foods.
Good sources: meats, poultry, ocean fish, tea, whole grains, and soft drinks (made in fluoridated-water areas)

HIGH-RISK GROUPS FOR POSSIBLE DEFICIENCY
- people living in areas with low-fluoride water content

RECOMMENDED DOSAGE
No RDA has been established .

GROUP	MG	GROUP	MG
Infants 0–0.6	0.1–0.5	Children 7–10	1.5–2.5
0.6–1	0.2–1.0	Young adults 11–18	1.5–4.0
Children 1–3	0.5–1.5	Adults 19 +	1.5–4.0
4–6	1.0–2.5		

TOXIC LEVELS
20 milligrams per day over long periods.

BENEFITS

TREATING DEFICIENCY SYMPTOMS
- dental caries
- osteoporosis

POSSIBLE BENEFITS
- protects against the breakdown of the bone of the jaw (a problem associated with a loss of teeth or following periodontal disease)

TOXIC SYPTOMS
Stained, deformed teeth and deformed bones.

DISCOVERY   Whether fluorine is an essential nutrient for humans is still a debated issue. As far back as the eighteenth century fluorine (or fluoride gas) was studied, and a French scientist, Henri Moissan, first isolated it in 1886. In the 1930s biochemists observed that communities with high fluoride content in their water supply had a much lower incidence of tooth decay. By 1945 the Public Health Service decided that adding sodium fluoride to the water supply was an effective and safe means of protecting a community against tooth decay. The now classic first study was conducted in Newburgh, New York, where 1 ppm (part per million) of fluorine was added to the water supply. In the following ten years children under the age of ten had 60–65 percent fewer DMF (the number of decayed, missing, and filled teeth) than another local community whose water was not fluoridated.

Over the years other long-term studies have shown continued and varied advantages of fluoridated water, including an extra protection against calcium loss that occurs during and following menopause.

ROLE   There is no specific metabolic function for fluorine, but as a structural component of teeth and bones, the protection it provides against dental caries is well documented. Recent studies suggested that fluoride also increases resistance to plaque acids on teeth.

PROBLEMS OF TOO LITTLE   A deficiency of fluoride in the diet increases the likelihood of dental caries, and it could possibly increase the risk of osteoporosis (see Calcium, page 150).

WHO IS AT RISK   No one.

TOO MUCH   Fluoride is a highly toxic element when consumed in excessive amounts; however, the fluorine content in water supplies in this country varies from .3 to 3.1 parts per million without causing any harm to humans. In those communities where the fluorine levels reach as high as 4 parts per million, fluorosis has appeared, which causes a brownish stain on the surface of the tooth and a pitting and roughening of the tooth surface.

STRATEGIES

FOOD SOURCES   Few foods contain more than 1 to 2 parts per million of fluorine. Since it is not an essential element for the life of plants, it usually is not present in any significant quantities in food from plants. Generally, meats, poultry, and ocean fish are dependable sources. Tea is also an extremely good source of fluorine, as is bonemeal when used as a mineral supplement. Normal drinking water provides from 1 to 2.5 milligrams per day in the average adult diet.

COBALT

DESCRIPTION
Cobalt's principal, if only, nutritional function is as an essential part of vitamin B12, or cobalamin. Therefore, cobalt is indirectly necessary for the prevention of pernicious anemia.

FOOD SOURCES
Meat and other animal foods.

HIGH-RISK GROUPS FOR POSSIBLE DEFICIENCY
• None.

RECOMMENDED DOSAGE
There is no recommended intakes for cobalt since there is no evidence of a cobalt deficiency for humans.

TOXIC LEVELS
High intakes of cobalt can cause a goitrogenic effect (goiters) and extensive intakes of cobalt chloride.

BENEFITS
None (other than that associated with vitamin B12; that is, cure of pernicious anemia).

DISCOVERY   Cobalt was discovered in 1742 by Swedish chemist Georg Brandt. For centuries it was used to make a deep blue pigment, but because the mineral resembled copper ore in some of its properties, the German miners named it *kobold* after an earth spirit because they believed this copper ore had been bewitched. By 1935 it was determined that cobalt was a trace element since it was found to be a constituent part of vitamin B12.

PROBLEMS OF TOO LITTLE   There is no known deficiency of cobalt since our diet provides on average about 3 milligrams and only .04 micrograms of that is required in vitamin B12.

MOLYBDENUM

DESCRIPTION
Molybdenum is a trace mineral that is an essential part of two enzymes which are involved in the mobilization of iron from the liver and in the oxidation of fats. It is also a factor in copper metabolism.

FOOD SOURCES
Meats, cereal grains, peas, and beans

HIGH-RISK GROUPS FOR POSSIBLE DEFICIENCY
- None.

RECOMMENDED DOSAGE

GROUP	MCG	GROUP	MCG
Infants 0–0.6	.03–.06	Children 7–10	.15–.50
0.6–1	.04–.08	Young Adults 11–18	.15–.50
Children 1–3	.05–.10	Adults 19 +	.15–.50
4–6	.06–.30		

TOXIC LEVELS
Have not been established.

BENEFITS
- None directly.

UNPROVEN BENEFITS (UNRELATED TO DEFICIENCY SYMPTOMS)
- prevents cancers
- prevents iron deficiency anemia
- builds healthy teeth

TOXIC SYMPTOMS

There is no human evidence of human toxicity, but laboratory studies suggest that it might produce diarrhea and poor growth and anemia.

DISCOVERY   In 1935 molybdenum was discovered to be an essential enzyme component, and this began the new area of research and discovery involving microelements or trace elements and enzyme action. The 9 to 10 milligrams of molybdenum found in the body is concentrated in the liver, kidneys, adrenal glands, and blood cells.

ROLE   Through its participation with the enzyme xanthine oxidase, molybdenum aids in the formation of uric acid from purines, a substance found in foods such as anchovies, kidneys, sardines, and sweetbreads. (Uric acid is the end product of purine metabolism, and it must be excreted because it cannot be destroyed within the body. Too much uric acid can cause gout.)

The enzyme also helps in the mobilization of iron from the liver reserves. The other enzyme, aldehyde oxidase, needs molybdenum for the oxidation of certain fats. Molybdenum may also help in the prevention of tooth decay by increasing the retention of fluoride. It is also thought to be a factor in copper metabolism.

PROBLEMS OF TOO LITTLE   The first actual case of a molybdenum deficiency was recorded in 1981, and it involved a surgery patient who was given an intravenous solution that was deficient in molybdenum and high in sulfur amino acids. The patient suffered from night blindness, mental disturbances, rapid heartbeat, and breathing problems. Eventually the patient fell into a coma, but when molybdenum was administered, the patient recovered. Molybdenum is now added to all parenteral (IV) nutrition solutions.

WHO IS AT RISK   No one.

TOO MUCH   Experimental evidence of molybdenum toxicity has produced symptoms such as diarrhea, poor growth, and anemia.

SELENIUM

DESCRIPTION
Selenium, along with vitamin E and the help of other enzymes, protect the cell against damage from toxic substances formed in the body called peroxides. Some other functions of selenium include the formation of connective tissue, and recent studies point to its involvement in the metabolism of the hormonelike substances "prostaglandins," fatty acid derivatives that are important in the regulation of many physiological functions. There is also a growing case made for a cancer-protection property of selenium.

FOOD SOURCES
Excellent sources: seafood (especially tuna and herring), kidney, liver, and other meats
Good sources: brewer's yeast, wheat germ, bran, whole grains, sesame seeds, egg yolks, mushrooms, chicken, milk, and garlic

HIGH-RISK GROUPS FOR POSSIBLE DEFICIENCY
- None.

RECOMMENDED DOSAGE

GROUP	MG	GROUP	MG
Infants 0–0.6	.01–.04	Children 7–10	.05–.20
0.6–1	.02–.06	Young Adults 11–18	.05–.20
Children 1–3	.02–.08	Adults 19 +	.05–.20
4–6	.03–.12		

UPPER LIMITS FOR REGULAR DIETARY SUPPLEMENT USE
For adults and children 7 years of age and older (for brief periods): .20 mg

TOXIC LEVELS
2.5–5.0 mg per day.

BENEFITS

TREATING DEFICIENCY SYMPTOMS
- abdominal muscle cramps following surgery

OTHER POSSIBLE BENEFITS
- complements vitamin E as an antioxidant
- promotes growth and development

UNPROVEN BENEFITS (UNRELATED TO DEFICIENCY SYMPTOMS)
- prevents and treats infertility
- slows the aging process
- cures cancer
- protects against cardiovascular disease
- protects against damage caused by smoking
- (with zinc) prevents hair from graying

TOXIC SYMPTOMS
First sign is a garliclike odor on the breath. Progressively, a loss of hair and nails, lesions of the skin, damage to the nervous system, and tooth decay.

DISCOVERY In his travels to China, Marco Polo reported the symptoms of a disease that we now believe was a selenium deficiency, but it was not until 1818 that the element was discovered by the Swedish chemist Jöns Jakobs Berzelius, who during his time was perhaps the greatest chemical authority in the world. The name selenium derives from the Greek *selene,* which means moon. There is no explanation as to why it was so named.

Animal researchers became interested in selenium in the 1930s when it was discovered that the grasses grown in some soils especially rich in selenium were actually toxic to grazing animals. The affected animals would grow stiff and lame. Ironically, in the 1950s biochemists learned that this same substance, in smaller quantities, could cure the ailments in animals that were a result of a vitamin E deficiency. From this experience biochemists soon discovered that the antioxidant properties of selenium were also essential to humans as well as cattle.

ROLE Found in minute amounts in the body, selenium is stored primarily in the liver and kidneys, containing four to five times as much as in muscle and other tissues. Selenium is normally excreted in the urine; if found in the feces, it is usually an indication of improper absorption.

Selenium is a key component in an extremely important enzyme called glutathione peroxidase. This is an antioxidant, which protects body tissues from the harmful effects of free radicals, which are very active molecules that damage cell tissue since they need other molecules with which to react. (Vitamin E is safer and equally as potent in this respect.)

Research on the question of selenium and cancer has produced evidence that suggests the distinct possibility that dietary selenium may be one of the many health factors that offer some defense against carcinogens. Results to date are unclear, however, because a study conducted in Oregon intended to demonstrate the relationship between blood selenium and breast cancer in women produced no such evidence. Another research study produced dietary liver necrosis, the death of liver tissue, in animals due to a selenium deficiency.

Some other functions of selenium include the formation of connective tissue, and as recent studies point out, it is involved in the metabolism of the hormonelike prostaglandins, fatty acid derivatives that are important in the regulation of many physiological functions.

Selenium may also favorably affect the heart muscle.

PROBLEMS OF TOO LITTLE   Selenium deficiencies are relatively rare in this country, but they have been recognized as a problem for some people. It is believed that a deficiency would adversely affect the heart since a chronic deficiency will enlarge the heart and impair its function. A disease that affects the heart muscle, Keshan's disease (named after a province of China where it is prevalent), is very common in parts of China where the soil and foods are selenium-poor. In other parts of the world, selenium-poor soil has been found to correlate with certain kinds of cancer.

WHO IS AT RISK   Only those people who eat food that comes primarily from soil that is selenium-poor. In such a place as Keshan, China, selenium deficiencies have affected hundreds of thousands of children and young women of childbearing age. In 1980 a study was published showing that the cause of the heart trouble in these children was a selenium deficiency that could be corrected with selenium supplements. New Zealand is another area of the world that is selenium-poor.

The only other people at risk might be those on parenteral (IV) nutrition solution since some of the reported cases of selenium deficiency have been hospitalized persons fed in this manner.

TOO MUCH   Since selenium is stored in the body and a toxic buildup can occur, doses should not exceed 250 to 500 micrograms daily and not for more than five days. Supplementation should never exceed 750 micrograms unless under the supervision of a physician.

An outbreak of selenium poisoning occurred in China in the 1960s when a local rice crop failed and inhabitants of five villages consumed vegetables from a region where selenium-rich coal contaminated the soil in which the vegetables were grown. Fifty percent of the villagers became seriously ill before the cause was discovered. In the United States there is no evidence that humans living in high-selenium areas develop symptoms attributable to dietary selenium. Because food nowadays comes from many different regions, human diets even in areas with high-selenium soil and water content almost never furnish more than .3 micrograms, which is a safe level.

It is speculated that high doses of selenium would cause such symptoms as loss of hair and nails, lesions of the skin, damage to the nervous system, and tooth decay.

STRATEGIES

FOOD SOURCES   The average diet may contain only 35 to 60 micrograms per day. The best food sources of selenium are seafoods such as tuna and herring. To a lesser extent selenium is also found in brewer's yeast, wheat germ, bran, whole grains, sesame seeds, egg yolks, mushrooms, chicken, liver, kidney, milk, and garlic (which accounts for its reputation for producing garlic breath). The selenium content of fruits and vegetables are relatively low, and they vary, as with all plants, because the selenium content of the food is determined by the content in the soil. For this reason the tables of selenium content of specific foods are highly unreliable.

FOOD PREPARATION   Appreciable losses of selenium can occur in the processing and cooking of food.

DRUG INTERACTION   Vitamin C taken with selenium will decrease its absorption.

CHROMIUM

DESCRIPTION
As a part of specific enzymes, chromium is involved in the metabolism of glucose for energy, insulin metabolism, and with protein-digesting enzymes in the intestine. Evidence points to the possibility that chromium plays a role in the synthesis of fatty acids and cholesterol in the liver.

FOOD SOURCES
Excellent sources: brewer's yeast, black pepper, and other spices, meats, (especially liver and kidney), oysters, and egg yolks
Good sources: whole wheat, salmon, nuts (including peanuts, walnuts, filberts, and Brazil nuts), mussels, and honey

RISK GROUPS FOR POSSIBLE DEFICIENCY
(No one group can be truly called "high risk.")
- people on a severe low-calorie diet
- people over the age of 60
- people with malabsorption disorders
- people with kidney disease
- pregnant and breast-feeding women
- people recovering from gastrointestinal surgery or severe burns
- people on long-term parenteral (IV) nutrition

RECOMMENDED DOSAGE

GROUP	MG	GROUP	MG
Infants 0–0.5	.01–.04	Children 7–10	.05–.20
0.5–1	.02–.06	Young Adults 11–18	.05–.20
Children 1–3	.02–.08	Adults 19 +	.05–.20
4–6	.03–.12		

TOXIC LEVELS
Have not been established.

BENEFITS

TREATING DEFICIENCY SYMPTOMS (THOUGH EXTREMELY RARE):

- diabeteslike symptoms
- weight loss
- nerve degeneration

UNPROVEN BENEFITS (UNRELATED TO DEFICIENCY SYMPTOMS)

- cures cancer
- treats arthritis
- prevents baldness
- prevents heart disease

TOXIC SYMPTOMS (ALTHOUGH RARE)

Skin problems, liver and kidney impairment, and lung cancer.

DISCOVERY   As early as 1797 a French chemist, Louis-Nicolas Vauquelin, discovered a new metal in a mineral from Siberia. Because of the many different colors in its compounds, it was named chromium from the Greek word *chroma,* which means color. Very early in this century biochemists learned that chromium existed in animal tissues, but it was not until 1959, ironically at the height of the craze for the oversized chrome-plated bumpers on American cars, that scientists at the National Institutes of Health discovered chromium was necessary in laboratory rats for normal metabolism of blood glucose. Seven years later it was officially associated with a human dietary deficiency. Since then, chromium has been known as the glucose tolerance factor.

ROLE   As with many microminerals, chromium's contribution to human nutrition is not fully understood, which makes it a continuing subject of much research. It is widely agreed, however, that chromium, combined with enzymes, is required for the optimal utilization of glucose and energy production. It is also believed that it helps to bind insulin to the cell so that glucose can be taken up by the cell. Less well understood, but also believed by researchers, is that it is somehow associated with one of the protein-digesting enzymes in the intestine.

PROBLEMS OF TOO LITTLE   In laboratory settings and in some chromium-poor parts of the world, deficiencies have been associated with poor glucose utilization and an increase in diabetes. Other symptoms associated with chromium deficiency are nerve degeneration, weight loss, retarded growth, and in some cases, heart lesions.

WHO IS AT RISK   Though deficiencies are rare, studies indicate that humans experience a steady decline through their life, which suggests to some researchers that the elderly may be at some, albeit small, risk of chromium deficiency.

Once again, people receiving parenteral (IV) nutrition are occasionally at risk of some nutritional deficiencies, and chromium can be one of them. Several hospitalized patients have developed an unexplained weight loss and diabeteslike symptoms while being fed intravenously. Once chromium was added to their diet, however, all the symptoms were reversed.

Those with a malabsorption disorder or kidney disease or recovering from gastrointestinal surgery or severe burns may have difficulty absorbing chromium.

TOO MUCH Chromium toxicity occurs principally, if not exclusively, as the result of inhaling contaminated air or drinking water containing excess amounts of the mineral.

STRATEGIES

FOOD SOURCES Like selenium, the amount of chromium in food is sharply dependent on the amount found in the soil. Foods that are good sources of chromium are brewer's yeast (and probably beer), fats (especially corn oil), and meats (especially liver and kidney), oysters, egg yolks, salmon, nuts (especially peanuts, walnuts, filberts, and Brazil nuts), mussels, honey, and black tea. Drinking water is also a primary source of chromium.

Fruits and vegetables are only fair sources, and fish is considered a poor source of chromium.

FOOD PREPARATION Information about chromium and foods is very limited. Studies have demonstrated that some of the mineral is leached out while cooking, but on the other hand, stainless-steel cooking utensils can contribute small amounts when acidic foods are cooked in them.

DRUG INTERACTIONS None.

NICKEL

DESCRIPTION

Nickel is found in the blood and in all human tissue, but its nutritional functions are not fully understood. One of its functions appears to be associated with DNA and RDA formation. In addition to being present in nucleic acids, nickel is thought to activate several enzymes and also interact in some manner with iron; for example, the symptoms of an iron-deficient diet are aggravated in the presence of nickel, but when iron levels are adequate, nickel appears to enhance iron utilization.

Nickel was discovered in 1751 by Swedish mineralogist Axel Fredrik Cronstedt. It was called Kupfernickel ("Old Nick's copper," in reference to the devil) because the miners believed that the metal was bewitched since it looked like copper but was not. Nickel is now more seriously viewed as a trace element because nutritional studies in the 1970s produced deficiencies in experimental animals. There are no known deficiency symptoms in humans, however.

VANADIUM

DESCRIPTION

Vanadium was identified in 1851 by Swedish chemist Nils Gabriel Sefström. Discovered during his studies of iron, Sefstrom named it vanadium after Vanadis, one of the names of the Norse goddess of beauty. For many years it was known to be present in plants and animals, but in 1970 experiments with chickens and then rats showed vanadium to be an essential trace mineral in these animals. Consequently, it is suspected that vanadium plays some kind of a role in growth, and probably with iron. It may also be associated with the metabolism of fats and the development of the bones.

Because vanadium requirements are so low (probably about .1 to .3 milligrams per day) and our diets contain about ten times that amount, human deficiencies are virtually unknown.

SILICON

DESCRIPTION

This trace element comes from the Latin word *silex,* which means flint. As an element it was discovered in 1824 by the same man who identified selenium, Jöns Jakob Berzelius. The results of animal studies in the 1970s provided the first evidence that silicon may be necessary for human growth. It is believed that it initiates calcification of bones, and it probably plays some role in the promotion of collagen formation.

The human requirement for silicon is not known but it must be small. The average diet contains more than enough for proper growth and health. (Beer has a high concentration of silicon.) This is one reason why the practice of taking silicon supplements for strengthening bones is unnecessary.

ARSENIC

DESCRIPTION

The most recent (1980) mineral to be considered essential for human nutrition is arsenic. The evidence is not conclusive, but minute traces of arsenic are found in plant and animal forms of life. Rats raised on arsenic-free diets exhibited slow growth patterns, and chickens and pigs seemed to benefit from arsenic added to their diet. Arsenic is believed to be an element of cell life and is present in eggs and seafood.

Arsenic is well known for its toxicity, and if taken orally will cause nausea, vomiting, diarrhea, dehydration, severe abdominal pains, and possibly death.

OTHER TRACE ELEMENTS

Three trace elements—tin, lead, and boron—are not widely considered as essential to human nutrition. They are found in some plant and animal tissues, however, and animal studies are yielding results that suggest a possible, though limited, nutritional role in animal life. As research develops we may learn more about their various nutritional functions, and in so doing, may come to reconsider their role in human nutrition.

TIN

DESCRIPTION

Tin is not found in the tissues of most animals or in newborn babies. (The fact that tin is found in adult tissue could be the result of contamination.) The results of one experiment conducted on rats in 1970 pointed to increased growth associated with tin.

There is little information about the tin content of food. It is thought that since acidic fruit juices can dissolve the tin from a tin-plated can, tin may be suitably represented in a diet that includes juices from unlacquered cans. This fact does not increase the likelihood of any toxicity since tin is not highly toxic. Generally speaking, our diet probably varies widely in the amount of tin it contains.

LEAD

DESCRIPTION

Lead is not thought of as a nutrient, and it is not, but rats fed diets that were deficient in lead did not grow to full size. Though there is no known metabolic role for lead, some researchers are studying its possible relationship to iron and copper.

Lead is obviously highly toxic, especially for children who have chewed on painted surfaces or toys that contain lead. Lead-glazed plates and dishes should not be used for food service. Lead will also appear in some water supplies because water is a good solvent for lead.

BORON

DESCRIPTION

Boron appears to be necessary for plant life but has no known role in the life and growth of animals. Researchers are looking into the possibility that boron affects the metabolism of calcium. Most people are familiar with the element boron as either boric acid or borax, neither one of which is found in food.

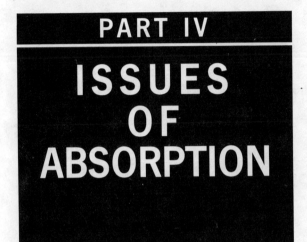

PART IV

ISSUES
OF
ABSORPTION

Absorption is the act of being swallowed or taken in. In this particular instance we will talk about how the body takes in the nutrients of the food we eat. We will also discuss the dynamics of digestion and metabolism because they are central to the entire discussion of nutrient absorption.

The word digestion is derived from the Latin *digestio,* which means to take apart, and the root meaning of the word metabolism is found in the Greek *meta,* which means change. Appropriately, the whole process of digestion and metabolism can be correctly described as a taking apart and change since the food we eat is prepared for absorption in our body through a process that removes from the food bulk the nutrients that cannot be absorbed, and changing them by forming with other substances to permit them to be successfully absorbed.

Absorption is an event that primarily takes place in the small intestine, but it is only the end result of the larger process called digestion. We will therefore begin the discussion of absorption with some facts about the digestive process: what happens, where it happens, and why it happens.

DIGESTIVE PROCESS

The distance food travels from the mouth to the anus is about thirty feet, and the total amount of time (from consumption to elimination) averages about twenty hours. During that time our food is shaped, chemically treated, absorbed into the bloodstream (directly or indirectly), and then finally its waste is eliminated. What is not absorbed, which is the indigestible, undigested, or unabsorbed food residues, is passed out of the body in the feces. In addition to these food residues, the feces consist of digestive secretions, mucus, dead cells from the lining of the gastrointestinal tract, bacteria, and water. Some residues from the metabolism of our foods are also passed out in the urine.

Digestion is both a chemical and a mechanical process. The mouth is where we break up and chew our food into small pieces and mix it with saliva. The saliva, which is secreted from three pairs of salivary glands located on each side of the face, contains a digestive enzyme, amylase, that begins the process of breaking down complex carbohydrates into simple sugars. (Protein and fats wait until the stomach before the chemical process of their metabolism begins.)

After the food is chewed and swallowed, it moves through the pharynx, where it is formed into a bolus or small lump, and then it moves down into the esophagus. The action that permits the bolus to move through the esophagus and into the stomach is called peristalsis, a series of wavelike muscular contractions.

In the stomach the food is mixed together with secretions of digestive enzymes and hydrochloric acid. These gastric chemicals begin to break down proteins and fats, and they continue the metabolism of the carbohydrates.

The next stop on this passage is the small intestine, which is a long tubular organ neatly coiled in loops about twenty-two feet long. It sits immediately below the stomach and is surrounded by the large intestine and colon. The food moves more easily into the narrow small intestines because by this time the gastric juices have turned the food into a thin liquid. Here, in the small intestine, most of the nutrients—minerals, vitamins, carbohydrates, lipids (fats), and proteins—are absorbed into the cells that line the digestive tract and from there directly into the bloodstream—or, in the case of some fats, into the lymph and then into the bloodstream. This is basically the end of the process for absorption of our foods.

The remaining mass, which is mostly fiber and water, continues through the ten feet of the large intestine where much of its water is absorbed, leaving a progressively more solid mass until it reaches the anus as semisolid fecal matter.

ABSORPTION This is a process by which products of digestion pass out of the small intestine into the cells of its lining and from there into the bloodstream or the lymph.

Nutrients such as simple sugars, amino acids, and some fatty acids are absorbed directly into the bloodstream from the lining of the small intestine; some large fatty acids are absorbed into the lymph system and then into the bloodstream.

Not all nutrients are absorbed into the body from the small intestine; for example, simple sugars as well as drugs can be absorbed in the mouth. Alcohol, which requires no chemical treatment for its absorption, finds its way into the bloodstream from the stomach. Minerals that need the presence of acids to be absorbed, such as iron and calcium, are absorbed in the upper part of the intestine, very near the stomach, where the acid medium is the strongest. For virtually all the other nutrients, especially lipids, proteins, and many carbohydrates, absorption takes place throughout the length of the small intestine.

Successful absorption requires cooperation. For many nutrients this means the assistance of a carrier substance, usually a protein, to carry them from the intestine to the bloodstream. The absorption of vitamin B12, for example, is dependent on a protein secreted by cells in the wall of the stomach, and the absorption of vitamin A depends on a single protein called a retinol-binding protein. Some proteins can carry a number of minerals, such as iron and manganese, and other proteins carry a whole group of fats, as in the case of lipoproteins.

The vitamin folacin (folic acid) needs an intestinal enzyme in order to be absorbed, while iron calls on the assistance of vitamin C (ascorbic acid) for its absorption. Iron absorption also gets a boost from highly acidic foods such as citrus juices, because iron needs an acidic solution for successful absorption.

Bile, a substance made in the liver and stored in the gallbladder, plays a role in absorption by enabling fats and fat-soluble vitamins, which are insoluble in water, to pass through the membrane lining of the intestine. Bile salts accomplish this feat by forming with carbon compounds to create a water-soluble compound that then binds with lipids for absorption. The principle is the same as that of dishwashing detergents that bind with greasy (fat) food residues in dishwater.

Issues of Malabsorption: Some dietary substances found in some foods can interfere with our absorption of nutrients. Fatty acids can bind with calcium and magnesium to form an insoluble compound that will impair absorption. Oxalic acid, found in spinach, rhubarb, and collard greens, will form an insoluble compound called calcium oxalate. Another substance found in the outer husks of whole-grain cereals, called phytic acid, will cause trouble by binding with calcium, iron, and other minerals to form a nonabsorbent compound. (See page 253 for table of Oxalate-Rich Foods.)

Other substances that meddle with absorption, specifically iron absorption, is the tannic acid of commercial black tea, the phosphates of some cheeses, and a substance called polyphenol in coffee. Even the form in which iron appears in our diet will determine the quality of its absorption; for example, the iron found in animal foods is called heme iron, and it is far more absorbent than the nonheme form of iron found in plant foods (see Iron, page 191).

Activities related to successful absorption almost never cease. Gastric enzymes are secreted into the stomach continuously, and the lining of the digestive tract is always being replaced. So if either of these functions is impaired or fails, absorption is immediately affected, sometimes seriously.

Malabsorption is also a matter of age. Over time the production of gastric acid is reduced, and there is a progressive degeneration of the intestinal tract.

One of the major signs of intestinal disorder is the malabsorption of nutrients, usually experienced as anemia. The cause of these disorders or diseases can be intestinal tumors, structural defects of the intestine, a failure to produce digestive enzymes, intestinal inflammation and infections, and gastrointestinal surgery. The body can also develop intolerances toward specific foods that make them unable to be absorbed; for example, a common disorder is lactose intolerance, which is caused by a lack of lactase, an enzyme secreted in the wall of the small intestine and needed to break down the sugar in cow's milk called lactose.

Another problem of malabsorption is celiac disease, an inherited disease that prevents the absorption of gluten, a protein found in wheat and rye. This disease is usually seen only in children, but some adults have been diagnosed with the disorder. As with any food intolerance or food allergies, the primary treatment is a diet that avoids those offending foods. If the problem of malabsorption is grave, steroid medications are used.

Many drugs, both prescription and over-the-counter, impair the value of many nutrients in our foods. In some cases we can be placed at risk of a specific deficiency if we take the drug for any period of time without supplementing our diet with more of the nutrient in question. For nutrients discussed in this book there is a list of those drugs that negatively affect their absorption or value.

Any one of these problems of digestion may initially appear to be only a nuisance, but if its symptoms persist, it can become a serious health problem. Whether it is diarrhea or nausea or excessive gas, if it continues for more than a few days, a physician should be consulted. If these symptoms are accompanied by fever and vomiting, especially if the patient is an infant, a physician should be consulted promptly.

As we have seen, digestion is an interdependent activity that requires the cooperation and presence of a variety of nutrients without which the process of absorption may be impaired. Overall poor nutrition may be only the result of a single deficiency since the lack of one nutrient can impair the utilization of virtually all the other nutrients. Good nutrition is, then, a matter of balance. Too much of one or too little of another can cause harm. Our diet should regularly draw from all four food groups to ensure that we enjoy all of the nutrients that work together for the sake of our good health.

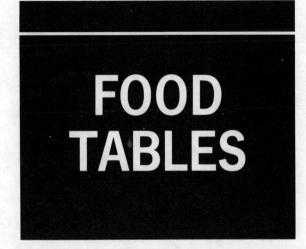

FOOD
TABLES

ACIDIC FOODS

Some foods produce an acid when metabolized that is important in the metabolism of other nutrients.

Bacon	Corn	Meat
Noodles	Crackers	Peanut butter
Brazil Nuts	Cranberries	Plums
Breads	Eggs	Poultry
Cakes	Fish	Prunes
Cereals	Lentils	Walnuts
Cheese	Macaroni	

ALKALINE FOODS

These foods produce alkali when broken down in the body. This alkali is excreted by the kidneys and contributes to the alkalinity of the urine.

Almonds	Cream
Buttermilk	Fruits (except cranberries, prunes, and plums)
Chestnuts	Milk
Coconuts	Vegetables (except corn and lentils)

CALCIUM-RICH FOODS

Calcium is essential for healthy teeth and bones. It is also needed for normal blood clotting and proper functioning of muscles, nerves, and cell tissue. Calcium is the one mineral that is the most deficient in our diet.

Food	Serving Size	Calcium (milligrams)
Almonds	1 cup	500
Brewer's yeast	15 tablespoons	500
Broccoli	2½ cups	500
Cottage cheese	12 oz.	500
Collard greens	1 cup	500
Custard	1 cup	500
Ice Cream	1⅔ cups	500
Milk: whole, low-fat, or buttermilk	8 oz.	500
Oysters	12 (approximate)	500
Salmon, canned with bones	5½ oz.	500
Sardines, canned with bones	3½ oz.	500
Soybean curd	8 oz.	500
Spinach	2 oz.	500
Yogurt	¾ oz.	500

CARBOHYDRATE FOODS, SIMPLE AND COMPLEX

Simple carbohydrates contain only calories ("empty calories"). Complex carbohydrates are rich in other nutrients that are important to good health.

Simple	Complex
Cakes	Beans
Candies	Breads
Cookies	Carrots
Corn Syrup	Cereals
Fruits	Corn
Honey	Crackers
Jams	Nuts
Molasses	Pasta
Soda	Peas
Sugar, maple	Potatoes
Sugar, table	Winter squash

CHOLESTEROL-RICH FOODS

Cholesterol is a waxy substance circulated through the blood system that is central to the production of cell membranes and substances such as hormones. It is also important to the protection of nerve fibers.

Food	Serving Size	Cholesterol (milligrams)
Bacon	2 oz.	33
Beef, cooked	4 oz.	94
Butter	1 tablespoon	31
Cheese, Brie	2 oz.	41
Cheese, cheddar	2 oz.	55
Cheese, processed	2 oz.	50
Cheese, creamed cottage	½ cup	5
Chicken, cooked	4 oz.	109
Cod, cooked*	4 oz.	68
Crab, cooked*	4 oz.	114
Cream, half-and-half	¼ cup	17
Egg	1 medium	220
Herring, cooked*	4 oz.	115
Lamb or pork, cooked	4 oz.	110
Liver, cooked	4 oz.	380
Lobster*	4 oz.	171
Milk, whole	1 cup	35
Salmon, smoked*	4 oz.	80
Sardines, canned*	4 oz.	114
Shrimp, cooked*	4 oz.	229
Sole, cooked*	4 oz.	68
Tuna, packed in oil*	3 oz.	55
Turkey, cooked	4 oz.	92

* These foods are rich in a fatty acid which possibly reduces the effects of dietary cholesterol.

DIETARY FIBER-RICH FOODS

Dietary fiber promotes good digestion and it also appears to reduce the likelihood of several gastrointestinal diseases. Since fiber is indigestible, it moves through the digestive tract unchanged and eventually moistens the stool and increases its bulk. It is believed that the fiber also speeds the passage of the feces through the colon, reducing the possibility of constipation, diverticulosis, and the development of cancer of the large intestine.

Food	Serving	Fiber (grams)
Apple, with skin	1 medium	2.0
Beans, baked	½ cup	7.3
Bran	½ cup	15.4
Bread, whole wheat	1 slice	.5
Broccoli, cooked	1 cup	4.1
Brussels sprouts, cooked	1 cup	2.9
Cabbage, cooked	¾ cup	2.1
Carrots, cooked	¾ cup	3.7
Cereal (All-Bran)	1 cup	19.0
Cereal (Grape-Nuts)	½ cup	4.7
Cereal (shredded wheat)	1 biscuit	3
Corn, cooked	1 ear	6.6
Corn, canned	½ cup	7.3
Orange, raw	1 medium	2.6
Peanuts, roasted	½ cup	5.8
Pear, with skin	1 medium	3.0
Peas, canned	½ cup	5.3
Pineapple, raw	1 cup	1.9
Plum, with skin	1 medium	1.4
Potatoes, baked	1	3
Prunes, with pits	5 large	8.0
Raisins	½ oz.	1
Spinach	½ cup	3
Strawberries	1 cup	3.3
Tomatoes, raw	1	2.0
Turnips, boiled	3 oz.	2.3
Walnuts	½ cup	3.0

FOLIC ACID-RICH FOODS

Folic acid (also known as folacin) is a B-complex vitamin that is needed for the manufacture of nucleic acids—RNA and DNA—the genetic material found in all cells. It is also required for the normal metabolism of amino acids, which are the building blocks of proteins.

Food	Serving Size	Folic Acid (micrograms)
Almonds	1 cup	136
Apple	1 medium	5–20
Bananas, raw	medium	26–33
Beans, green	1 cup	20–50
Bread	1 slice	5–15
Brewer's yeast	1 tablespoon	100–150
Broccoli	2 stalks	100–150
Carrot	1 medium	5–20
Cheese, hard	1 oz.	5–20
Cucumber	1 small	20–50
Egg	1 large	20–50
Garbanzo beans	1 cup	300–400
Liver	3 oz.	100–150
Milk	8 oz.	5–12
Mushrooms	3 large	5–20
Orange juice	6 oz.	100–150
Potato	1 medium	5–20
Soybeans, dry	1 cup	300–360
Shellfish	6 oz.	20–50
Spinach	4 oz.	100–170
Yogurt	8 oz.	20–50

FAT COMPOSITION OF COMMONLY USED FATS AND OILS

Saturated fats increase blood cholesterol levels, while polyunsaturated fats and monounsaturated fats decrease blood cholesterol levels.

Food (1 tablespoon Polyunsaturated serving)	Saturated (grams)	Monounsaturated (grams)	Polyunsaturated (grams)
Butter	9	5	trace
Coconut oil	11	1	trace
Corn oil	2	4	7
Margarine			
hard (vegetable oils only)	5	7	2
soft (vegetable oils only)	5	6	3
Peanut oil	3	7	4
Olive oil	2	10	2
Safflower oil	2	2	11
Sesame oil	2	5	5
Soybean oil	2	4	8
Sunflower oil	2	5	7

GOITROGEN-RICH FOODS

Goitrogens are substances that bind to iodine and thus prevent it from being available to the thyroid gland for the production of thyroid hormones (see table of Iodine-Rich Foods, page 250).

Brussels sprouts	Cauliflower	Rutabagas
Cabbage	Kale	Soybeans
Carrots	Peaches	Spinach
Cassava (tapioca pudding)	Pears	Turnips

IODINE-RICH FOODS

The thyroid gland needs iodine to enable it to produce the thyroid hormone thyroxine, which controls the rate at which the body's cells function, as well as the rate of growth and the development in children.

Food	Serving Size	Vitamin D (mcg.)
Baked goods	3 oz.	9
Cheese	2 ozs.	8
Egg	1 medium	7
Kelp	3 oz.	36
Meat	4 oz.	20
Milk	1 cup	34
Salt, iodized	1 gram	74
Seafood	4 oz.	62

IRON-RICH FOODS

Iron is crucial for the formation of hemoglobin, which carries oxygen in the blood. It also increases resistance to stress and disease.

Food	Serving Size	Iron (milligrams)
Apricots, dried	6 large halves	2
Beans, lima	1 cup	4
Beef, lean	3 oz.	5
Bologna	3–4 oz.	1.5
Bread	1 slice	7
Brewer's yeast	1 tablespoon	2
Broccoli	1 cup	1.2
Carrots	1 cup	0.8
Chicken, all cuts	3–4 oz.	2
Collards	1 cup	1.8
Cream of Wheat	1 cup	1.4
Eggplant	½ cup	0.7
Fruits, including: apples, bananas, cherries, melons, citrus, pineapple, etc.	1 piece	1
Lamb, lean	4 oz.	5
Liver, calf's	1 oz.	4.0–5
Molasses, blackstrap	1 tablespoon	2.0–4
Mushrooms	⅓ cup	.3–.7
Oatmeal	1 cup	1.5–2
Pasta	½ cup	.3–.7
Peanut Butter	2 tablespoons	.3–.7
Peas, cooked	½ cup	2.0–4
Pork, fried	1 slice	24
Potato	1 medium	1.4
Pumpkin seeds	2 tablespoons	1.5
Raisins	½ cup	4
Rice, cooked white or brown	1 cup	1.5

MAGNESIUM-RICH FOODS

Magnesium is responsible for releasing energy from the food we eat. It is also important for muscle contraction and for proper blood calcium levels.

Food	Serving Size	Magnesium (milligrams)
Almonds	1 oz.	75
Apples, raw, unpared	medium	50
Avocado	3 oz.	40
Bran	1 oz.	140
Cashews	1 oz.	75
Cereal, whole grain	1 oz.	40
Cheese	2 oz.	25
Chocolate	2 oz.	170
Hazelnuts	1 oz.	50
Lima beans, cooked	1 oz.	90
Peanuts	1 oz.	50
Pecans	1 oz.	40
Pistachios	1 oz.	45
Shrimp, cooked	4 oz.	60
Soybean curd	3 oz.	95
Spinach, cooked	1 cup	110
Walnuts	1 oz.	40
Wheat germ	1 oz.	100

NIACIN- (VITAMIN B3–) RICH FOODS

This vitamin is found in all cells of the body and is essential to providing energy for their growth. It is also important to the metabolism of carbohydrates.

Food	Serving Size	Niacin (milligrams)
Asparagus, cooked	1 cup	1.9
Beef	4 oz.	5.9
Bread, whole wheat	1 slice	.8
Chicken	4 oz.	8.0
Corn, sweet	1 cup	2.5
Lamb	4 oz.	5.7
Liver, cooked	4 oz.	18.2
Peanut butter	1 tablespoon	2.5
Peas	1 cup	3.2
Pork	4 oz.	5.7
Potato, broiled	1 medium	1.6
Rice, long-grain	1 cup	2.1
Swordfish, cooked	4 oz.	11.4
Tuna, canned	3 oz.	12.7
Turkey	4 oz.	8.0
Veal	4 oz.	8.0

OXALATE-RICH FOODS

Oxalates are organic substances found in some foods. If taken in large enough quantities, Oxalates will bind with calcium to form kidney stones in susceptible people.

Beans, baked	Grapes	Spinach
Beans, green	Kale	Squash, summer
Beets	Lemon peel	Strawberries
Blueberries	Parsley	Tangerines
Celery	Peppers, green	Tea
Chocolate	Raspberries	Watercress
Collard greens	Soybean curd	Wheat germ
Eggplant		

PHOSPHORUS-RICH FOODS

Phosphorus helps in building strong teeth and bones, the transference of nerve impulses, the contraction of muscles, and the release of energy from carbohydrates, fats, and protein. Phosphorus is abundant in our diet.

Food	Serving Size	Phosphorus (milligrams)
Almonds	1 oz.	130
Apricots, dried	3 oz.	100
Brains, cooked	4 oz.	400
Bran	1 oz.	260
Brazil nuts	1 oz.	170
Cereal, whole grain	1 oz.	95
Cheese	2 oz.	165–430
Chocolate milk	3 oz.	120–200
Fish, cooked	4 oz.	145–600
Kidneys, cooked	4 oz.	400
Liver, cooked	4 oz.	200
Milk	1 cup	225
Peanuts	1 oz.	100
Peas, cooked	1 cup	85
Walnuts	1 oz.	145

POTASSIUM-RICH FOODS

This nutrient is essential for the proper functioning of all muscle contraction, especially the heart, for the metabolism of carbohydrates and proteins, and for transmitting nerve impulses in the brain and throughout the body. Along with sodium, potassium also regulates the amount of water in the individual cell.

Food	Serving Size	Potassium (milligrams)
Avocado	1	1,836
Banana	1 medium	560
Beans, Lima	1 cup	724
Brussels sprouts, fresh cooked	1 cup	950
Carrots, cooked	1 cup	344
Chicken, broiled	6 oz.	483
Clams	3 oz.	225
Dates, pitted	10	518
Flounder	6 oz.	1,000
Milk, skim	1 cup	406
Orange juice	1 cup	496
Potato, baked	1 medium	782
Prunes, dried and pitted	5 large	298
Spinach, raw	1 cup	1,600
Sweetbreads	3 oz.	433
Tomato, raw	1 small	250
Tuna, salt-free, canned	3½ oz.	327
Yogurt, plain	1 container	531

RIBOFLAVIN- (VITAMIN B₂-) RICH FOODS

Vitamin B_2 (riboflavin) breaks down proteins, fats, and carbohydrates into energy. It is necessary for the growth and repair of cell tissues throughout the body, especially of the skin, mucous membranes, and the eye.

Food	Serving Size	Vitamin B_2 (milligrams)
Asparagus	½ cup	.12
Beef, lean roast	4 oz.	.25
Broccoli	⅓ cup	.13
Brussels sprouts	½ cup	.11
Cheese, creamed cottage	½ cup	.30
Chicken	4 oz.	.21
Collard greens	½ cup	.19
Egg	1 medium	.16
Ham	4 oz.	.21
Hamburger	4 oz.	.24
Lamb, leg of	4 oz.	.31
Liver, beef	4 oz.	4.8
Milk, 2% fat fortified	1 cup	.52
Milk, skim	1 cup	.43
Milk, whole	1 cup	.41
Sardines	4 oz.	.23
Spinach	½ cup	.11
Squash, winter	½ cup	.15
Tuna, canned	3 oz.	.12
Veal, roast	4 oz.	.35
Yogurt	½ cup	.22

SELENIUM-RICH FOODS

The primary function of selenium, along with vitamin E, is to protect the cells against damage from toxic substances called peroxides that are formed in the body.

Food	Serving Size	Selenium (milligrams)
Beef kidney	3 oz.	90–150
Beef liver	3 oz.	17–68
Bread, rye	3 oz.	18–34
white	3 oz.	15–36
whole wheat	3 oz.	32–46
Cheese, American	3 oz.	71
Chicken liver	3 oz.	56–70
Fish, cod	3 oz.	21–39
herring	3 oz.	52
lobster	3 oz.	19–38
mackerel	3 oz.	56
oysters	3 oz.	24–56
sole	3 oz.	13–25
tuna	3 oz.	75–120
Ham	3 oz.	28–44
Lamb	3 oz.	15–38
Milk, skim	1 cup	12
Milk, whole	1 cup	3
Molasses	3 oz.	50–150
Peanuts	3 oz.	33
Pork sausage	3 oz.	17–58
Rice, brown, dry	3 oz.	34
Rice, white, dry	3 oz.	6–30
Salami	3 oz.	17–60

TYRAMINE-RICH FOODS

Tyramine-rich foods cause severe migraine headaches among susceptible people.

Alcoholic beverages (especially sherry;
   beer; and Chianti, Reisling,
   and sauterne wines)
Bananas
Bologna
Broad Beans
Cheese, aged
Chocolate
Eggplant
Figs, canned
Fish, dried
Herring, pickled
Hot dogs
Liver (chicken and beef)
Meat tenderizers
Pepperoni
Pickled herring
Pineapple
Plums
Salami
Soy Sauce
Yeast and yeast extracts
Yogurt

VITAMIN A-RICH FOODS

This vitamin is needed for the health of the skin, and it is believed to be necessary for a healthily functioning immune system. The proper growth of teeth, hair, and eyes depend upon vitamin A, as do bones and glands.

Food	Serving	Vitamin A (I.U.)
Apricots, dried	6 halves	2,500
Asparagus	½ cup	600
Beans, green	½ cup	340
Broccoli	½ cup	2,360
Cantaloupe	½ cup	6,500
Carrots	½ cup	7,600
Egg	1 medium	600
Liver, beef	4 oz.	60,500
Milk, whole	1 cup	350
Orange juice	½ cup	270
Peach	1 medium	1,320
Peas, green	½ cup	430
Potato, sweet	½ cup	8,500
Pumpkin	½ cup	8,200
Squash, winter	½ cup	4,300
Tomato juice	½ cup	970
Yogurt	½ cup	340

THIAMIN- (VITAMIN B1-) RICH FOODS

Vitamin B1 (thiamin) is needed to break down carbohydrates into glucose, for the maintenance of nerve tissue, and in the promotion of appetite. The vitamin is found in red blood cells, the liver, and the kidney.

Food	Serving Size	Vitamin B1 (milligrams)
Asparagus	½ cup	.11
Beans, dried	½ cup	.13
Beef liver	4 oz.	.31
Cereal	½ cup	.10
Collard greens	½ cup	.14
Ham	4 oz.	.55
Lamb, leg of	4 oz.	.17
Lima beans	½ cup	.16
Milk, 2 percent fat fortified	1 cup	.10
Orange juice	½ cup	.10
Oysters	¾ cup	.25
Pork, lean roast	4 oz.	1.25
Rice, enriched	½ cup	.12
Spaghetti, enriched	½ cup	.10
Veal, roast	4 oz.	.15

PYRIDOXINE- (VITAMIN B6-) RICH FOODS

Vitamin B6 (pyridoxine) is needed for amino acid metabolism, the formation of certain proteins, and the proper functioning of the nervous system.

Food	Serving	Vitamin B6 (milligrams)
Bananas	1 medium	.60
Beef, cooked	4 oz.	.30
Cabbage, cooked	1 cup	.12
Carrots, cooked	1 cup	.10
Fish, cooked	4 oz.	.23–.95
Grape-nuts cereal	3 oz.	2.41
Liver, cooked	4 oz.	.83
Milk	1 cup	.10
Oatmeal	1 cup	.30
Peanuts	1 cup	.58
Pork, cooked	4 oz.	.45
Potato, baked	1 medium	.28
Veal, cooked	4 oz.	.34

COBALAMIN- (VITAMIN B12-) RICH FOODS

Vitamin B12 is needed for the normal development of red blood cells and for the healthy functioning of all cells, particularly those in the bone marrow, nervous system, and intestines.

Food	Serving Size	Vitamin B12 (micrograms)
Beef, cooked	4 oz.	1–2
Cheese	2 oz.	.7
Chicken, cooked	4 oz.	1.0
Egg, cooked	1 medium	.8
Fish, fatty, cooked	4 oz.	5–30
Lamb, cooked	4 oz.	1–2
Liver, cooked	4 oz.	28–121
Milk	1 cup	.8
Pork, cooked	4 oz.	1–3
Veal, cooked	4 oz.	1.1
Whitefish, cooked	4 oz.	1–5

VITAMIN-C RICH FOODS

Vitamin C (ascorbic acid) is needed for the production of collagen, a protein necessary in the formation of connective tissue in skin, muscles, blood vessels, bones, and cartilage. It also contributes to the health of teeth and gums, aids in the body's absorption of iron, and in healing wounds.

Food	Serving Size	Vitamin C (milligrams)
Broccoli, cooked	1 cup	120
Brussels sprouts, cooked	1 cup	140
Cantaloupe	½, 5-inch diameter	63
Cauliflower, cooked	1 cup	66
Collard greens, cooked	1 cup	87
Cranberry juice	1 cup	81
Grapefruit juice	1 cup	102
Kale, cooked	1 cup	68
Lemon juice	1 cup	110
Orange	1 medium	60
Orange juice	1 cup	50
Parsley, raw, chopped	1 cup	68
Papaya	1 cup, cubed	102
Pepper, raw green	1 cup	95
Pineapple juice	1 cup	80
Spinach, cooked	1 cup	50
Strawberries	1 cup	85

VITAMIN D-RICH FOODS

The major function of this vitamin is to regulate calcium and phosphate metabolism, which is necessary for the development of healthy, strong teeth and bones.

Food	Serving Size	Vitamin D (I.U.)
Egg, cooked	1 medium	28–36
Herring, broiled	4 oz.	1,000.0
Liver, calf's, cooked	4 oz.	11.4
Milk	1 quart	400.0
Salmon, canned	3 oz.	428.6
Sardines, canned in oil	3 oz.	257.0
Tuna, canned in oil	3 oz.	199.0

VITAMIN-E RICH FOODS

Vitamin E has an important role in protecting our cell and membranes from wear and tear (see Selenium, page 217). It also appears to be helpful in the healing of burns and wounds when topically applied.

Food	Serving Size	Vitamin E (milligrams)
Almonds, raw	1 oz.	7
Cod liver oil	1 tablespoon	3
Corn oil	1 tablespoon	12
Olive oil	1 tablespoon	2
Peanuts, raw	1 oz.	6
Pecans, raw	1 oz.	8
Safflower oil	1 tablespoon	5
Sesame seed oil	1 tablespoon	4
Soybean oil	1 tablespoon	15
Soybeans, dry	3 oz.	17
Sunflower seed oil	1 tablespoon	10
Walnuts, raw	1 oz.	6
Wheat-germ oil	1 tablespoon	35

VITAMIN K-RICH FOODS

Vitamin K is needed for the manufacture of certain substances in the liver responsible for blood-clotting.

Food	Serving	Vitamin K (micrograms)
Asparagus, cooked	1 cup	83.0
Bacon, cooked	2 oz.	26.3
Bread, whole wheat	1 slice	4.8
Broccoli, cooked	1 cup	310.0
Cabbage, cooked	1 cup	87.5
Cheese	2 oz.	20
Lettuce	1 outer, 2 inner, 3 heart leaves	29.4
Liver, beef, cooked	4 oz.	104.9
Oats, rolled	1 cup	48
Spinach, cooked	1 cup	160.2
Turnip greens, cooked	1 cup	942.5

ZINC-RICH FOODS

Zinc is needed in digestion and metabolism. It is essential to the growth and development of reproductive organs. Insulin relies on zinc to function properly, and this mineral also affects the absorption of vitamin A.

Food	Serving Size	Zinc (milligrams)
Apple sauce	1 cup	.5
Beef, lean	3½ oz.	5.0
Bran	¾ cup	1.0
Bologna	3–4 oz.	1.5
Bread, white	2 slices	1.0
whole wheat	2 slices	1.5
Cheese, cheddar	1 oz.	.1
Chicken breast	3 oz.	1.0–1.5
Clams	3 oz.	1.0–1.5
Egg	1 medium	.5
Lamb	3½ oz.	4.0
Liver	3 oz.	4.5
Milk, whole or skim	8 oz.	.7
Oysters, Atlantic,	3½ oz.	75.0
Pacific	3½ oz.	9.5
Pineapple juice	8 oz.	.4
Pork, lean	3½ oz.	4.5
Potato, cooked	1 medium	.5
Rice, brown	1 cup	1.0
white	1 cup	.5
Tomato	1 medium	.5
Tuna	3 oz.	1.0
Wheat germ	1 tablespoon	1.5

INDEX

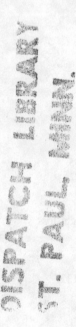